G000111568

The Slow Poisoning of America

John E. Erb
T. Michelle Erb

Paladins Press

COPYRIGHT 2003 BY JOHN AND MICHELLE ERB
All rights reserved. No part of this book may be reproduced without permission of the publisher.

ISBN: 0-9741993-0-3

PUBLISHED BY

PALADINS PRESS

VIRGINIA BEACH, VIRGINIA.
www.spofamerica.com

This book is dedicated to our wonderful children with the hope that they will live in a world that is happy, healthy and safe.
Thank you for inspiring us to fulfill our duty as parents to offer you the best world for you and your children to inherit.

A special debt of gratitude goes to the scientists, researchers and free thinkers that we have made reference to in this book. Thank you to those who have asked the questions, without fearing the answers.

Table of Contents

Rude Awakening

From the look on her face I could tell that something terrible had happened. "What is it?" I asked her. Her voice trembled as she spoke, "It's our daughter, she's been poisoned."

Shock hit me. How could we, middle class, well-educated parents, have allowed our daughter to be poisoned? When our children came into this world, we wrapped them in the security of our arms. Holding them close we made promises that no harm would ever come to them as long as we stood guard.

How could this happen? Under our watchful eyes our daughter had developed a case of poisoning. Would our daughter survive?

"What poisoned her, should we call poison control, 911? What is it, what can be done about it?"

"There's nothing we can do. Jessi has Fluoride poisoning."

I was dumbfounded and confused. Fluoride? The wonder chemical that we grew up believing would protect us from cavities? Fluoride, which politicians and dentists proclaimed to be so good for our health that it was added to our water supply? How was it possible that such a beneficial additive could poison our 6 year old?

"How can you tell, what makes you think Jessi's poisoned?" I asked, not believing for a moment what Michelle was saying. She must be over-reacting to something she read or saw on TV.

"Look at her teeth." Michelle replied. "See for yourself. The white mottled marks on her new teeth that are just coming in, take a close look."

I went to the family room where Jessi was happily tracing a pony in one of her favorite coloring books.

"Hi Sweetie, could you smile for me and show me your pretty new teeth?"

Jessi, always quick to show off her radiant smile, happily obliged. I took a close look, closer than I'd ever had before. Sure enough, just as Michelle had said, the new teeth sprouting in her mouth were mottled with what looked like abnormal white patches. I thanked her for her smile and returned to Michelle.

"Okay, her teeth look a little abnormal, but what makes you think it has anything to do with fluoride poisoning?"

Michelle wasted no time dragging me over to the computer.
"I noticed the spots a few days ago," she said, "and decided to see what it was." On the monitor was a very large picture of a child's mouth, filled with mottled white teeth. Underneath it was the caption: Dental Fluorosis caused by Fluoride Poisoning.

I was shocked and dismayed. I was not yet willing to believe that for years I have been not only brushing with, but also drinking poison. I finally allowed myself to relax a little. "Michelle, it doesn't look so bad, it's just little blotches on her teeth. Poisoning, you say? I think you're overreacting."

Michelle had always known I was a hard sell, a hard-line believer in 'government knows best' ideology. Having worked in local government offices, and having faith in the absolute truth of mass media news, I was in no hurry to side with my wife's radical claim. Jessi was a very healthy, pretty little girl. She was already taller and larger than any of her classmates. I honestly felt my wife's claims were unfounded. Had I known then what I know now, I would have seen the foolishness of my ways.

Michelle, never being one to give up easily, fell to work gathering the data that she would use to try to win me over to her line of thinking. She scoured the Internet, local libraries and bookstores.

In between amassing supporting evidence, we took Jessi to a dentist. We had recently moved so the dentist that had seen her previously was not available. The new dentist took one look at Jessi and supported Michelle's diagnosis. He said it was Dental Fluorosis. When asked the cause the dentist replied that it was from Jessi getting too much fluoride when her permanent teeth buds were forming. He said that some children eat the toothpaste, and get too high a dose. Will it go away on its own, we asked? The dentist replied that it was irreversible. He said that when Jessi gets older, there are some treatments that would make the damage less noticeable. The dentist tried to make us feel better by adding that we shouldn't worry, 30% of children now have dental fluorosis, and Jessi's case wasn't even considered severe.

The visit to the dentist made me feel a little better, knowing Jessi was not at death's door and that she was among a large group of children, not just a single victim. The news only acted to make Michelle angrier. She was deeply hurt by the fact that the dentist we had seen when Jessi was four told us that we needed to give her fluoride-fortified water. The dentist also said she needed a fluoride rinse. Like good parents we listened to the dental professional and blindly followed the regimen prescribed. Little did we know that the added fluoride had created the case of poisoning we now saw before us.

Michelle would not sit idly by accepting the consolations of the dentist. She went to her reference sources. The whole question of fluoride opened before her like a giant jigsaw puzzle. One by one, she uncovered the pieces and one by one she put them into place. The final scene that lay before us was more frightening, more threatening and more far reaching than we could have ever imagined.

Sodium Fluoride, the popular drinking water additive, has been widely used as rat poison.

The facts were uncovered and the truth was clear. Jessi had been poisoned, poisoned by the dentists that promoted the fluoride treatments, poisoned by the companies that made the toothpastes, poisoned by the cities that fluoridate the water, and most importantly, poisoned by the government that promoted fluoride for its own questionable reasons.

I had finally seen enough.

The plethora of articles, news releases, books and web sites that Michelle inundated me with broke through my indoctrinated brain.

The fog lifted from my mind and I was able to see clearly the institutional and governmental system that was actively denying and burying the facts of the dangers of fluoride.

If you have any doubt as to the dangers of fluoride, look on the back of the toothpaste tube that your children use. The paste is flavored like bubble gum or candy to ensure that children use large gobs of the stuff. If you live in the United States you will see the words: Warning: there is enough fluoride in this tube to seriously harm a small child. If a larger than pea size amount is swallowed, call poison control.

What will poison control tell you? Fluoride is a highly toxic chemical. It is more poisonous than lead, and only slightly less toxic than arsenic. The governments of both United States and Canada have done their best to ban lead. It is no longer in gasoline, or in paint, and houses that have lead paint must declare a warning to the buyer. On the other hand Fluoride, a tube of which can kill a small child, is found on every grocery store shelf in America, flavored to attract even the most fussy of children. Worse still, the governments of United States and Canada advocate the adding of fluoride to almost every city water supply in their nations.

Today, with all our wisdom and technology, governments are purposely adding something more toxic than lead to the water that we give to ourselves, our children, even our babies.

Michelle was right.

The mounting evidence was inarguable, especially for as die-hard a scientific thinker as myself. We had poisoned our daughter with fluoride. The American and Canadian Dental Association, and the federal governments themselves, supported and extolled the virtues of this poison. We had unwittingly fallen prey to their rhetoric and propaganda. Why would the government promote the use of one of the most toxic substances? What could governments gain by poisoning their own people? Worst of all, if these governments who we trust with our health and safety lie about the dangers of fluoride, what other secrets are they hiding? What other substances that the politicians regard as safe and beneficial, could actually be harmful, even deadly to people, especially to our children?

With this concern in mind, Michelle and I were determined to research as much as possible about every substance our children eat, drink, and breathe. Through determination and diligence, the list of dangers that we discovered grew. Fluoride was just a drop in the bucket. Soon we discovered an entire rogue's gallery of chemicals suspected in causing everything from blindness to cancer. All of these items shared one thing in common, the governments of United States and Canada allow them to be used unchecked and without warning to consumers.

No matter the consequences.

Fluoride, Supposed to be Good for You

I still remember when we took Jessi to the dentist for the first time. She was three years old, with a head full of curly blond hair. Her baby teeth shone pearly white, smiling as she skipped into the office. She couldn't wait to show the dentist her pretty teeth. In the office the staff doted on her Shirley Temple charm. We stood by her side as the dental hygienist fussed over her.

When the dentist came in, we told him about our concern. Jessi had a severe intolerance to dairy products. A mouthful of milk or cheese would send her stomach into convulsions, and send us running for a bucket. How was she to get her calcium? Would her bones and teeth be strong and healthy? No problem, the dentist told us. When she is older she will get fluoride treatments, to help protect her fragile teeth. We left the office with a smile and a new toothbrush, trusting in the wisdom and benevolence of the health professional.

Little William may also have been smiling when his mother took him to the Brownsville Dental Health Center in Brooklyn. He was only three years old and it was his first visit to the dentist. Mrs. Kennerly was likely pleased when Dr. George announced that her son didn't have a single cavity. She was probably relaxed when Ms. Cohen, the dental hygienist came into the room. Ms. Cohen used a swab to spread fluoride gel over William's small teeth. While chatting with a co-worker, Ms. Cohen handed William a cup of water. She didn't tell him to rinse and spit; so three year old William drank it down.

William immediately started vomiting, sweating and complaining of headache and dizziness. Five hours later, he slipped into a coma and died. William was the victim of fluoride poisoning.

The date was May 24, 1974.[1]

Almost thirty years later, we still haven't learned. In dentist's chairs all over North America, the scene is repeated over and over. Parents everywhere step back and put their trust in dental staff, who proceed to spread a toxic treatment of sodium fluoride in their child's mouth.

Remember the warning on the toothpaste tubes that states that swallowing a pea size amount of it can cause toxic reactions?

The gel that the dentist puts on your child's teeth can be 20 times more toxic then toothpaste. Now remind your child not to swallow, even though the five-minute wait to take the poison off may seem like forever.

Even after the dental treatment ends, your child is still at risk from the fluoride. Dr. John Yiamouyiannis, author of Fluoride and the Aging Factor, reports that up to 6% of children who receive fluoride treatment at the dentist's office complain of side effects like nausea and vomiting within an hour of receiving the fluoride treatment.

How did it come to this? When did we as parents forget our vow to protect our children from harm and agree to have a highly toxic substance smeared in their mouths? Is the fear of dental cavities so strong that we resort to poisoning our children and ourselves?

The dental profession has made us fear cavities. Parents all over North America are having their children brush with fluoride, sometimes three times a day. We are buying fluoridated

---

[1] "$750,000 Given in Child's Death in Fluoride Case: Boy, 3, Was in City Clinic for Routine Cleaning" **New York Times**. January 20, 1979.

mouthwash. We are supporting fluoride toothpaste programs in our schools. Some children are even prescribed fluoride tablets.

Thousands of cities across the U.S. and Canada have water supplies that are already polluted with fluoride. Thousands more actually pay for fluoride to be added to their public water supply.

In the name of reducing cavities, we have turned our water supply into a flowing medical prescription that we have not been given the choice of participating in.

How was a toxin like fluoride turned into a universal treatment for cavity prevention?

The history of the fluoride lie is as shocking as the damage it does to your children.

Fluoride began receiving scientific recognition in the 1920's. Parts of United States and Canada had become so heavily industrialized that air and water pollution was becoming an issue. Large refineries were smelting iron, copper, steel and aluminum. Towering brick smoke stacks belched out millions of tons of hazardous gases. The smelting process left behind contaminated wastewater, which was poured into the rivers, lakes and streams.

In 1920's, dentists became aware of mottled chalky white areas developing on children's teeth. It was determined that the aberrations were caused by fluoride in the drinking water so the scientists called the problem Dental Fluorosis. Dentists at the time were disgusted by the occurrence of fluorosis, and wanted fluoride to be removed from the water supply altogether.[2]

Big business had other ideas.

Enter on the scene, Andrew Mellon. Mellon had a problem that needed to be solved. Andrew Mellon had founded the incredibly successful Aluminum Company of America (ALCOA). The

---

[2] Groves, Barry Fluoride: Drinking Ourselves to Death. Gill and Macmillan 2001, page 179

process of aluminum smelting creates large amounts of the liquid bi-product sodium fluoride. With the new pressures against polluting, and the fear of fines and penalties, Mellon had to find a solution to the huge amounts of sodium fluoride collecting on his properties.

Andrew Mellon was in a very unique position. From the late 1920's to the 1930's, he not only owned the aluminum company, but was also the Treasury Secretary for the United States Federal government. Conveniently enough, the U.S. Public Health Service (USPHS) was under the jurisdiction of Mellon's office.

In 1928, Dr. Frederick McKay observed that teeth that had fluorosis may be more resistant to cavities.[3] Mellon took an interest in fluoride's affect on teeth and, in 1931 had H. Trendley Dean of the USPHS study the water supplies. Dean determined that as fluoride levels increased in water, so did the amount of fluorosis on teeth. He continued his research and in the late 1930's, Dean published purposely skewed data to show that a concentration of 1 part per million gallons in water, fluoride produced a minimal amount of dental fluorosis and resulted in the reduction of tooth decay."[4]

Dr. Gerald Cox, a biochemist on staff at the Mellon Institute (founded by the Mellon family in 1913 to advance science and industry) made a public proposal that 1ppm was the optimal level of fluoridation in water. He suggested that any community whose water was less than this solution should be bolstered with more fluoride. His proposal likely received support from big industry because it created a way to rid themselves of fluoride. If fluoride could be shown to be good for people, than it could be dumped into the rivers straight from the factories.

The most effective way to get rid of a toxic substance would be to package it as a beneficial health additive. Of course, you would have to get the roach and rodent poison makers to stop writing

---

[3] McKay, F.S. Relation of Mottled Enamel to Caries. J Am Dent Assoc 1928: 15: 1429-37.

[4] Yiamouyiannis, Dr. John. Fluoride: The Aging Factor. Health Action Press 1993, page 141.

Sodium Fluoride on the sides of their packaging. Not to worry, with enough marketing people won't notice that rat poison and the dental wonder drug are one and the same.

It baffles my mind that people could believe the following argument: "Arsenic is poisonous to people, but if we give them a little everyday; it will be good for them." This argument is identical to that of those supporting fluoride.

Luckily, even in the 1930's and 40's, there were people who saw the dangers of fluoride. In 1931, both the "American Dental Association and the U.S. Public Health Service called for the removal of fluoride from waters where it naturally occurred and from air where it was found as a result of industrial contamination."[5]

The editor of the Journal of the American Medical Association, and the editor of the Journal of the American Dental Association wrote scathing reviews on fluoride in water.

"Fluorides are general protoplasmic poisons,......the sources of fluorine intoxication are drinking water containing 1 part per million or more of fluorine.....another source of fluorine intoxication is from the fluorides used in the smelting of many metals, such as steel and aluminum." **Journal of the American Medical Association 1943**[6]

The American Medical Association's editorial specifically stated that fluoride intoxication occurs at 1 part per million, the same level that the government now promotes. The AMA also identifies the source of this poison to be aluminum mills like the ones Mellon owned.

A far more effective argument about the dangers of fluoride came in 1944 from the American Dental Association:

---

[5] Yiamouyiannis, Dr. John. Fluoride: The Aging Factor. Health Action Press 1993, page 140.

[6] "Editorial: Chronic Fluorine Intoxication", **Journal of American Medical Association**, Volume 31, pp 1360-1363 (1943).

"We do know the use of drinking water containing as little as 1.2 to 3.0 parts per million of fluorine will cause such developmental disturbances in bones as osteosclerosis, spondylosis and osteopetrosis, as well as goiter, and we cannot afford to run the risk of producing such serious systemic disturbances in applying what is at present a doubtful procedure intended to prevent development or dental disfigurements among children." **Journal of American Dental Association**[7]

With both the American Medical Association and the American Dental Association sternly objecting to the presence of fluoride in drinking water, why is it that in 1952, and even to this day, these same organizations support its use?

Political pressure.

Andrew Mellon, owner of ALCOA and the corporate mind behind fluoridation, died in 1937. He had been disgraced as the U.S. Treasurer whose policies helped begin the Great Depression. Even after his death, his mission to find a home for his company's toxic waste lived on.

In 1944 Oscar Ewing arrived to carry on Mellon's quest to find a home for aluminum's mounting toxic waste. Ewing was an attorney at Mellon's Aluminum Company of America, pulling in questionable salary of $750,000 a year (that would be about 8 million in today's funds). He suddenly left that position to take a dramatic pay cut and become Federal Security Administrator. As such he was in charge of the United States Public Health Service.[8]

With assistance from Edward Bernays, nephew of Sigmund Freud and author of the 1928 book *Propaganda*, Oscar Ewing manipulated popular opinion to make the opponents of fluoridation look like 'crack pots and right wing loonies.'[9]

---

[7] "Editorial: Effect of Fluorine on Dental Caries," **Journal of American Dental Association,** Volume 31, pp 1360-1363 (1944).

[8] Yiamouyiannis, Dr. John. Fluoride: The Aging Factor. Health Action Press 1993, pg 142.

[9] Griffiths, J. "Fluoride: Commie Plot or Capitalist Ploy" **Covert Action,** Number 24, pp 26-29, 63-66. (1992).

Oscar Ewing managed to convince a few dentists to promote fluoride, and in 1945 a pilot project was started in Grand Rapids Michigan that would test the success of water fluoridation. The study was to last ten years, with recommendations about fluoride's effectiveness reported to the government after the study's completion. The administrator of the study was Trendley Dean, the USPHS researcher of questionable repute when Andrew Mellon was in charge of things.

But the ten year long study was never completed. Ewing's propaganda machine had been set in motion and by 1946, only one year after the Grand Rapids experiment began and before any facts supporting fluoride, was in full swing.

Advertisements read: "ALCOA sodium fluoride is particularly suitable for the fluoridation of water supplies........If your community is fluoridating its water supply – or is considering doing so – let us show you how ALCOA sodium fluoride can do the job for you."[10]

In 1947, two years after the start of the Grand Rapids experiment, six more U.S cities and 87 more towns opted to fluoridate their water. Their municipal governments were now poisoning thousands of Americans. Pandora's box had been opened; to close it now would be to welcome disaster to fluoridation's promoters and risk the litigation of the governments that supported it.

In 1950, five years before the study of the Grand Rapids project was to be completed, both the United States Public Health Service and the American Dental association suddenly announced their endorsement of water fluoridation. Even though the gathered data to date did not show enough evidence in favor of the project, the USPSHS started promoting countrywide fluoridation. In 1951, Frank Bull, Director of Dental Education for the Wisconsin State Board of Health, gave a speech at the Washington Conference of

---

[10] **J Am Water Works Association** 1950. 43 – 6.

State Dental Directors on how professionals in the industry should promote fluoride:

"Now in regard to toxicity...the term adding sodium fluoride. We never do that. Sodium fluoride is rat poison. You add fluorides. Never mind that sodium fluoride business...if it is a fact that some individuals are against fluoridation, you have just got to knock their objections down. The question of toxicity is on the same order. Lay off it altogether. Just pass it over. 'We know there is absolutely no effect other than reducing tooth decay,' you say and go on."

Proceedings of the Fourth Annual Conference of State Dental Directors with the public Health Service and the Children's Bureau, Federal Security Building, Washington, DC, USA 6-8 June 1951.

Bull must have been an excellent orator, for to this day, the American Dental Association website 'www.ada.org', sticks to its convictions saying that though children's teeth may be permanently tainted with fluorosis, it is worth the risk to reduce cavities.

Permanent disfigurement, condemned in the ADA journal of 1944, is now welcomed by today's ADA as the price of a reduction in cavities.

Today over 80% of children in communities with fluoridated water have teeth visibly discolored by the toxic effect of fluoride.[11] Compare that rate to 0% in communities with no fluoride in their drinking water. Where would you want your children to live?

When your son or daughter smiles for a photo on their wedding day, look at their mottled, disfigured teeth, and breath a collective thanks to those brave folks at the ADA, CDA and the U.S. Public Health Service that promoted the poisoning of your child for life.

What about the arguments that fluoride reduces tooth decay?

---

[11] "Toxicological Profile for Fluorides, Hydrogen Fluoride, and Fluorine", **U.S. Public Health Service,** 1993.

To date, the studies arguing this benefit are flawed in both their methods and conclusions. Dr. John Yiamouyiannis, doctor of biochemistry and past president of the National Health Federation, did an exhaustive study of the dental data of 39,207 children from all over the United States. He examined the records of dental examinations completed under contract for the U.S. Public Health Service from 1986-1987. The studies included 84 areas with children ranging in age from 5-17. Of these areas, 30 had never received fluoridation in the water, 27 had only been partially fluoridated or fluoridated for less than 17 years, and 27 had been fluoridated for 17 years or more. He measured the average number of Decayed, Filled, and Missing Teeth (DFMT) per child.

By comparing the data, he found that the amount of DMFT per child held no relation to whether the community was partially, fully, or non-fluoridated. 543 students in non-fluoridated Buhler Kansas had the lowest rate of DFMT, at 1.23 per child. The next lowest city was fluoridated El Paso Texas, where 451 students had 1.32 DFMT. At the high range of the study, partially fluoridated Concordia County in Louisiana had 424 students with 3.77 decayed, missing and filled teeth per child. The non-fluoridated State of Hawaii had the second highest statistics, with the 293 students tested showing 3.29 DFMT.

The frequency of non, partially, and fully fluoridated communities was spread evenly on the DFMT results listing, supporting Dr. Yianouyiannis' conclusion that fluoridation has nothing to do with reduction in tooth decay.[12]

Barry Groves, in his book Fluoride: Drinking Ourselves to Death, pointed out that Germany, Austria, Denmark, Finland, Sweden, Norway, the Netherlands, Switzerland, France, Italy, Belgium, Hungary, Portugal, Greece, Japan, and China don't approve fluoride's addition to their water supplies. "It is only in countries in which the law makes fluoridation mandatory, or discussion of fluoridation illegal, that fluoride is widely used."[13]

---

[12] Yiamouyiannis, Dr. John. Fluoride: The Aging Factor. Health Action Press 1993, pg 127.

[13] Groves, Barry Fluoride: Drinking Ourselves to Death. Gill and Macmillan 2001, pg 227.

If the addition of fluoride to our water isn't benefiting our children, and ourselves, what is this poison doing to our bodies?

Here is what fluoride has been proven to do:

Fluoride is a rat and cockroach poison: Since the start of the century, companies have been marketing and selling sodium fluoride to effectively kill cockroaches, rats, and other vermin in homes across United States and Canada. Even as recently as 1987, a woman in Virginia died after ingesting sodium fluoride packaged as a roach poison.[14]. Let us not forget William Kennerly, the three year old who may have been alive today if it were not for fluoride.

Fluoride is the cause of fluorosis in teeth: Scientists have noted an association between mottled enamel and fluoride exposure since the early 1900's.[15]

When you look at the mottled white on your children's teeth you can blame fluoridation for that. The American Dental Association implies that it is worth a lifetime of esthetically displeasing teeth when you consider the value of the reduced amount of cavities you will get as a child.

The first evidence that fluoride has poisoned a child is when their permanent teeth begin to erupt around age 6. It is these teeth that show the extent to which fluoride has poisoned the child. The amount of white patches and ridges on the teeth directly shows the extent of the damage. This is only the visible damage; the other damage that fluoride does is hidden beneath the skin.

The ADA suggests that the problem is only cosmetic.

---

[14] Poklis A, Mackell MA. "Disposition of fluoride in a fatal case of unsuspected sodium fluoride oisoning." **Forensic Sci Int** 1989 Apr-May; 41(1-2):55-9.

[15] Bowen, WH. "Fluorosis: is it really a problem?" **J Am Dent Assoc**, 2002 Oct;133(10):1405-7.

Long after your child's teeth have surfaced the effects of fluoride poisoning, the toxic chemical continues to affect the hidden organs, tissues and bones within your body.

In India fluoride has been found at high levels in the water supply of several villages. People living there age abnormally. Many have arthritis and bone problems in their 30's. It was discovered that fluoride poisoning is the cause:

> *"The early symptom is the discoloration of teeth or what doctor's call 'mottling.' With the advancement of age, the teeth fall out giving the appearance of old age, followed by pain in the joints, hips and loss of flexibility."*[16]

The dangers of sodium fluoride are well documented. For those of you who work on a job site that uses any kind of chemicals, you may be aware that OSHA guidelines demand that a Material Safety Data Sheet be on site to explain the dangers, and the first aid treatment, of any chemical used on the job. Sodium fluoride is a common material used in a variety of industrial applications. Below is an excerpt taken directly from a standard MSDS used for Sodium Fluoride:

Sodium Fluoride EMERGENCY OVERVIEW

Appearance: white to off-white crystalline powder.

*Danger! Moisture sensitive. This substance has caused adverse reproductive and fetal effects in animals. **Harmful if swallowed**. May cause **lung damage**. Causes digestive and respiratory tract burns. May cause severe respiratory tract irritation with possible burns.*
Causes eye and skin irritation and possible burns. May cause severe digestive tract irritation with possible burns.

Target Organs: Kidneys, heart, gastrointestinal system, skeletal structures, teeth, nerves, bone.

---

[16] 'Relief illusive as life is crippled.' **The Hindu.** January 24, 1982.

Potential Health Effects:

Eye: Causes eye irritation and possible burns. May cause chemical conjunctivitis and corneal damage.

Skin: Contact with skin causes irritation and possible burns, especially if the skin is wet or moist. May cause skin rash (in milder cases), and cold and clammy skin with cyanosis or pale color.

*Ingestion: Ingestion of large amounts of fluoride may include salivation, nausea, vomiting, abdominal pain, fever, labored breathing. Exposure to fluoride compounds can result in systemic **toxic effects on the heart, liver, and kidneys.** It may also deplete calcium levels in the body leading to hypocalcaemia and death. May cause irritation of the digestive tract and possible burns. May cause respiratory paralysis and cardiac arrest.*

Inhalation: May cause severe irritation of the respiratory tract with possible burns. Aspiration may lead to pulmonary edema. Prolonged exposure to dusts, vapors, or mists may result in the perforation of the nasal septum. May cause systemic effects.

*Chronic: Chronic inhalation and ingestion may cause chronic fluoride poisoning (**fluorosis**) characterized by **weight loss, weakness,anemia**, brittle bones, and stiff joints. May cause **reproductive and fetal effects**. Effects may be delayed. Chronic exposure may cause **lung damage**. Laboratory experiments have resulted in **mutagenic effects**. Chronic exposure to fluoride compounds may cause systemictoxicity. Skeletal effects may include bone brittleness, joint stiffness, **teeth discoloration**, tendon calcification, and osterosclerosis. Animal studies have reported the development of **tumors**.[17]*

Workers who are exposed to sodium fluoride are educated in its dangers, now you are too. Perhaps every bathroom cabinet should have a Material Safety Data Sheet about fluoride attached to it.

How does this affect you? You don't work with Sodium Fluoride in a factory, why should you fear the effects outlined in this Safety Sheet?

Sadly, you come in contact with this poison everyday, in almost every fashion listed on this safety sheet.

---

[17] Acros Organics, Sodium Fluoride MSDS Chemical Product information sheet.

Skin: When you brush your teeth with fluoridated toothpaste, the sodium fluoride comes in contact with your skin, mouth, tongue and gums. This can cause acne-like skin eruptions.[18] It may be the cause of canker sores and other ailments of the mouth.

Ingestion: Small amounts of sodium fluoride are swallowed every time you or your child brushes with fluoridated toothpaste. The dangers of this prompted the FDA to place a mandatory warning label on each tube of toothpaste that contains fluoride.
This warning reads *"If you accidentally swallow more than used for brushing, seek professional help or contact a poison control center immediately."* The FDA also states that fluoride should not be given to children under the age of three due to its toxic effects. What is their reason for giving it after three? Does the poisonous effect of sodium fluoride disappear when a child reaches three? Or is it expected that at three children are over a certain weight, so that the toxic effects are distributed and diluted over a larger mass. Do we ever outgrow our toxic reaction to lead or arsenic? Why would we outgrow our intolerance to sodium fluoride?

Sodium fluoride has been reported to cause death in people when it is in doses of 1.2 grams or more.[19] The American Dental Association may argue that to get that amount of fluoride you would have to drink 1,200 litres of water fluoridated at 1 ppm. They fail to mention that a tube of toothpaste usually has 1,000 ppm of fluoride, and that the topical paste used by dentists may have up to 20,000 ppm. At those levels, one liter (4 cups) of dental office gel would have 20 grams of toxic sodium fluoride, enough to possibly kill 16 mature adults. Only 62 ml, or ¼ cup of this dental fluoride paste could kill an adult. So when the dental hygienists smear this flavored toxic paste on your child's teeth, stand back and relax, after all, your child knows enough not to swallow it, right?

[18] Saunders, Milton A. "Fluoride Toothpastes: A cause of Acne-like skin eruptions", **Archives of Dermatology**, Volume 111, p 793 (1975).
[19] Toth, K. "The role of fluorides in the prevention of dental caries" **Fogorv Sz** 1990 Jun; 83(6): 163-7.

The American and Canadian Dental Associations feels that the levels of fluoride in toothpaste are safe and well regulated. However, this is not the case. The FDA limits the amount of fluoride that can be put into toothpaste to no higher than 1150 ppm. In a letter to Mark Reuben, (CEO of the Colgate Palmolive Company) dated May 4th, 2001, the FDA cited his company on adding an extra 6 pounds of fluoride to one batch of Colgate toothpaste. Although the company laboratory tested the batch and found it to be outside the acceptable safe limits, the toothpaste was sent out for distribution anyway. If you used Colgate toothpaste in 2001, you may have exposed yourself and your children to fluoride far in access of what the FDA considers to be safe amounts. The FDA went on to point out in the letter that from 1998-1999, 12 lots of fluoride additive were not checked for levels of purity. This was a concern to the FDA because Colgate Palmolive does not certify its suppliers; the sources of the toxic additive are not fully investigated. Considering that one of the main suppliers of fluoride for use in toothpaste is the aluminum smelting industry and the fluoride could come directly from one of these industrial sites, it is important to know just what kind of other contaminants could also be in it.

These are only the violations noticed by FDA investigators during a weeklong visit to the Colgate site. What happens in the Colgate plant the other 51 weeks of the year?

Chronic: This kind of exposure occurs every time you drink from a fluoridated water supply. If you live in a fluoridated community, you ingest it every time you brew your coffee, or make a drink for your children. Every bottle of formula you make could have a dose of toxic sodium fluoride for your baby's delicate stomach.

Fluoride being added to water has been the cause of hundreds of poisonings in American cities. In a Mississippi town, families suffered gastrointestinal illness due to a malfunction in the fluoridation equipment that caused an increase of fluoride in the water to forty times its safe limits.[20]   Residents in an Alaskan community suffered much worse. 296 people fell ill from fluoride poisoning. They suffered "nausea, vomiting, diarrhea, abdominal pain, or numbness or tingling of the face or extremities." One of these victims even died.[21]   Once again, failure of monitoring and control of the public water system was blamed for the poisoning.

Sadly, the government response to this mass poisoning consisted of a simple suggestion that officials should watch the water system more closely. In both cases of fluoride poisoning in public water systems, it took several days for the authorities to realize it. In that time many people were needlessly poisoned. If you live in a fluoridated community, how safe do you feel knowing that a tank of toxic poison is attached to your public water supply, that at any moment, human or mechanical error can send large amounts of it streaming through the pipes into your home? You need not worry; the authorities are closely monitoring the situation, and may warn you three days after a toxic spill occurs.

What about those agencies meant to protect us from poisons? Surely the FDA and the Environmental Protection Agency would act to protect us from this danger?

The FDA knows that sodium fluoride is toxic. They have even gone so far as to ban it from being added to food. According to the FDA it is illegal for a company to add even a drop of fluoride to the foods you eat, yet it is added to something even more vital: the water you drink.

The EPA's public stand on water fluoridation is to promote it. Behind the scenes, however, the people who work within the EPA have another view.

The National Treasury Employees Union Local 2050 represents the 1500 scientists, lawyers, engineers and other professional

---

[20] Penman, AD. Brackin, BT. Embrey, R. "Outbreak of acute fluoride poisoning caused by a fluoride overfeed, Mississippi, 1993." **Public Health Rep** 1997 Sep-Oct;112 (5):403-9.

[21] Gessner, BD. Beller, M. Middaugh, JP. Whitford, GM. "Acute fluoride poisoning from a public water system". **N Engl J Med** 1994 Jan 13;330 (2):95-9.

employees at the EPA headquarters in Washington. This union took the stand that not only is water fluoridation poisonous, but that it should immediately be terminated. This demand comes directly from the people within the EPA itself; those with the inside scoop on the hazards of the poison that their Directors support.

A document titled *Why EPA Headquarters' Union of Scientists Opposes Fluoridation,* dated May 1st, 1999, and prepared on behalf of the Union Chapter Senior Vice President, J. William Hirzy, outlines the EPA employees stand with absolute clarity.

The Union document states that the employees at the EPA headquarters in Washington believed in the value of water fluoridation until 1985, when one of their scientists was pressured by management to make a false statement supporting the safety of fluoride in water if the limits were raised to 4mg/liter 4ppm. It was reported that the increase of allowable levels was demanded of the EPA by outside political forces. Perhaps by industries hoping to increase the allowable pollution limits? The demand by management for an EPA scientist to support fraudulent statements raised concern within the employees at the EPA. They started researching the side effects of fluoride in the drinking water. The EPA Headquarters employees union made the following startling discoveries:

➤ Human's brains and kidneys are being damaged with the 1 part per million dosage of fluoride they currently get in the water supply.

➤ Doses of fluoridated water can cause neurotoxic effects like hyperactivity.

➤ Fluoridated water can lead to a drop of 5-10 IQ points in children.

➤ Fluoridated water can reduce the pineal gland's ability to produce the hormone Melatonin; thereby disturbing sleep patterns and also quickening the onset of puberty in children.

➢ Fluoridated water increases the occurrence of the cancer Osteosarcoma.

➢ Fluoridated water causes skeletal fluorosis, leading to an increase of incidence of bone fractures in communities with this water treatment.

➢ Applied Fluoride (toothpaste and gels) can cause gene mutations and cancerous tumor growth.

The EPA employees were very concerned by these findings. Things between union and management became more heated when Dr. William Marcus, Chief Toxicologist of the Office of Drinking Water, was fired from the EPA for refusing to remain silent about the cancer risks of water fluoridation.

The greatest revelation is this: The EPA employees have discovered that water fluoridation has no beneficial ability to protect children from getting cavities. The union document cites studies of 39,000 children that show that there is no difference in frequency of caries (cavities) between children in fluoridated and non-fluoridated cities, (just as Dr. Yiamouyiannis stated) and that the only difference between the children in these two groups is that the children drinking fluoride show a higher chance of exhibiting destructive dental fluorosis.

Why is it that the employees of the government recognize the dangers of fluoride, yet the administration both at the EPA and at the U.S. Public Health Service promote it? Why are the top levels of government agencies ignoring their own experts by promoting fluoride?

Perhaps it's due to the CYA phenomenon. CYA, better known as 'Cover Your Ass' is a term being utilized by politicians and industry everywhere. It is the practiced art of covering up one's own mistakes, especially if those mistakes could lead to widespread lawsuits with the total discrediting and possible bankruptcy of those involved.

Imagine if the truth about the fluoride dangers came out. If the agencies promoting fluoridation would finally accept the true findings of the hundreds of scientific studies that prove the toxicity of sodium fluoride. If only the management at the EPA actually listened to its 1500 employees regarding the dangers of fluoride. If people everywhere stopped swallowing the government's lies about fluoride, what would happen?

People would ask why such a thing could happen in the first place.

How was it that a politician such as Andrew Mellon could, in his role as Treasury Secretary, sponsor studies that would make the toxic sodium fluoride that his own company (ALCOA) created, appear a positive thing for people?

How could Oscar Ewing, ALCOA employee and Director of the Federal Security Administration, manage to push through an experiment to fluoridate water that proved no conclusive evidence of its benefit?

How was it that the American Dental Association that once demanded fluoride be removed from water, suddenly promote its widespread use?

How is it that industries are being allowed to fill the sky and the rivers with sodium fluoride?

How could the government itself be involved in a cover up of epic proportions designed to hide poisons in the sheep's clothing of public health? Why is it that we are being poisoned for the sake of corporate profit?

These questions and more would demand answers. Boards of inquiry would be created. Politicians would be held accountable. Corporate records would be subpoenaed. Industries, which pollute the air and waters with fluoride, would face massive clean up fines. The ADA and its member dentists could face a class-action lawsuit that could crumble the entire dental industry.

The current government would rather support a flawed status quo than face the wraith of a deceived public. To admit that fluoride is a poison would be to declare half of the drinking water in America unsafe. The entire sodium fluoride program was the brainchild of ALCOA to dispose of its pollution. ALCOA continues to have a controlling interest in the Bush administration. 70 years after ALCOA's founder was Treasury Secretary for the U.S., Paul O'Neil, recent past president and CEO of ALCOA, became the Secretary of the Treasury under George W. Bush. While he was Secretary of the Treasury, O'Neil remained on the ALCOA payroll, receiving $926,000 a year in pension from ALCOA, which is considered to be one of the biggest polluters in Texas.[22]

The cost of treating community water supplies with either distillation or reverse osmosis to remove the fluoride would be enormous. The cost to industries to clean up the toxins they have poured into our waters would eat into their profits. Why allow the truth to come out, when the status quo is so much cheaper? What does it matter if children are poisoned, as long as industry and government stays in the black?

It is unfortunate that many politicians today do not support the clear thinking of Dr. A.L. Miller, U.S. representative from Nebraska. Chairman of the Special Committee on Chemicals in Foods. In 1952 he stated before Congress :

"I am a former state health director and have always supported the Public Health Service in the measures that they advocated. I am sorely disappointed that they now are advocating every single soul in the community should take fluoride before all the facts of experiments now in progress have been completed.
"Mr. Speaker, it is disturbing to me when the men in the Public Health Service, who, as late as 1950, were not ready to endorse the universal use of fluorine, have now, almost to a man, come out for the endorsement.

---

[22] Moore, Michael. <u>Stupid White Men</u>. HarperCollins New York 2001. Page 18.

"It is difficult for me to understand how high officials in the Public Health Service could change their mind, over a 3-month period and completely reverse the field. Where once they advocated for the go-slow sign on the use of fluorides they now apparently have gone overboard, and put out large amounts of propaganda favoring the fluoridation of water. I am certain that the dental profession merely echoes and endorses the opinions of the Public Health Service. They have done little experimental work themselves.

"Mr. Speaker, despite my best efforts, and from the evidence before my committee, I cannot find any public evidence that gave me the impression that the American Medical Association, the American Dental Association, or several other health agencies, now recommending the fluoridation of water, had done any original work of their own. These groups were simply endorsing each other's opinions.

"You will note that all of the experts grounded in the science of biochemistry have advocated the go-slow sign on the use of fluorides in drinking water. I believe that the dental profession and other like-minded individuals, like myself, have been misled by the Public Health Service, because all of the facts have not been made upon this subject......"

"I sometimes wonder if the Aluminum Company of America and its many subsidiary companies might not have a deep interest in getting rid of the waste products from the manufacture of aluminum, because these products contain a large amount of fluoride."[23]

If the U.S. Public Health service has, as Miller states, misled us all about the benefits of fluoride, our very faith in government would be shaken to its deepest foundations. If the government has lied about fluoride, what else are they lying to us about?

Fluoride is just the beginning.

---

[23] Miller, A.L. "Fluoridation of Water - Extension of Remarks" **Congressional Record**, March 25th, 1952, pp A1899-A1901.

Food Additives, the Good, the Bad, and the Ugly

Michelle and I have five children. Like other parents, we have tried to do everything possible to raise them in a healthy environment. Despite our best efforts, our children suffer from disorders that are now commonplace in the youth of the nation. Our thirteen year old was diagnosed with asthma; our twelve year old has fluoride poisoning and Attention Deficit Disorder; our eight year old has fluoride poisoning and a severe dairy intolerance; and our youngest, at seven, has been diagnosed with asthma and Attention Deficit Hyperactive Disorder.

Four out of our five children have been diagnosed with disabilities that can make life extremely difficult. Three of these children were prescribed costly medications that could have been a lifelong treatment.

How many of your children are in a similar situation? I am sure you ask yourself: "Where did I go wrong? Why is the healthy bundle of joy I brought home from the hospital not so healthy anymore? What can I do to make them well again?" These questions and more plague us. Every single day these thoughts cross our minds as we watch our children puff from an inhaler, or swallow their daily dose of Ritalin.

Not a day goes by that we don't wish we could take away all their ailments. What could we do differently that could have protected our children? Why are kids today, even with all our advanced technology, less healthy than the generations that came before?

The answer is simple: We poison them.

Every time we open a package of luncheon meat, we poison them.

Every time we heat up a can of soup, we poison them.

Every time we order at a fast food restaurant, we poison them.

Every time we hand them a diet soda, we poison them.

Every time we hand them a toothbrush, we poison them.

We poison them just a little each day and after a while, their little bodies start breaking down. ADHD, asthma, juvenile diabetes, gastric intestinal disease, obesity, allergies, and worst of all cancer. Children are being diagnosed with these illnesses in record numbers.

How did it come to this? When did we, the protectors of our children, suddenly become the harbingers of disease? It is a tragedy many years in the making. It started when we as parents stopped making the foods that our children put into their bodies. It started when companies began mass-producing prepackaged food for our consumption. It started when governments allowed known toxins to be added to foods under their approving eye. It started when we placed our trust in government and industry to put our children's health ahead of profit.

It will only end when YOU decide it does.

We devote ourselves, as all parents do, to giving our children the best of everything. Dress them in the best clothes, send them to the best schools and feed them with the best foods.

When it came to cooking for our children, we dove into the task with gusto. When we could afford it, we used the premium brands in our recipes: Kraft, Campbell's, Knorr and Bovril.

The times that we could not afford these trusted labels, we would hope that the less known brands would give our children almost as much nourishment as their higher priced counterparts. Surely the more expensive priced items used better ingredients to make tastier and healthier dishes.

For years we ladled out our tuna casserole, tacos, chicken fajitas and French onion soup, hoping that our homemade creations would rival the nutrition of the finest restaurants. Little did we know that our faith in the premium products was ill advised and unsubstantiated.

What we didn't know then is that the cans, boxes and packets of the majority of products that we made for our children's lunches, snacks and dinner whether brand name or no name, had more to do with consumer addiction than nutritional value.

As parents, we know how hard it is to get children to eat. They seem to get fussier with every passing generation. The garden grown cabbage and home made stews that my mother would place on the table would not pass the discerning palate of today's child.

What parent today has time to make a home baked apple pie, or pack a lunch made with bread from his/her own oven. Today's corporate world demands that parents to spend more time thinking about their finances or situations at work and less time worrying about what to put in their children's lunch boxes. In schools across America, fewer and fewer children are opening their brown bags to discover a home made meal. More and more of them are pulling out a mass produced item spewed from a well-oiled machine, prepackaged and portion controlled for convenience.

Parents defend themselves: 'I know it must be good for them because it says on the label, LOW SODIUM, LOW IN FAT.'

What companies forget to mark on the label is 'LOW IN FOOD VALUE, HIGH IN ARTIFICIAL INGREDIENTS.'

To prove this point, go into your kitchen and take out one of those prepackaged lunches that you are going to send in your little one's lunch or snack tomorrow. Look at the ingredients list. Count how many ingredients have names that you don't recognize. Many of these names sound like they could be found sitting in a pharmaceutical warehouse, or stirred into a laboratory petrie dish: Disodium EDTA, BHA, Propylene Glycol, Caseinate, Dimethyl Sulfate, Sodium Nitrate, to name only a few.

Just what are these substances? I have never seen any of them in the baking section of a grocery store. My grandmother never added them to her soups, bread, or pasta dishes. My mother never added them to my sandwiches, or her fresh baked apple pie. So what are they doing in the food we are giving to our children?

Open any recipe book you have on your shelf, you will not see a single recipe that calls for any of these items. Not a single cup, tablespoon, teaspoon or even pinch of these items are mentioned. What are they doing in the brand name foods that we trust to base our children's nutrition upon?

These man-made chemicals have a reason for being in the items you purchase, but it's not nutritional value. The reason manufacturers add these chemicals: Profit.

A tasty and attractive product sells, a product that can last for months before it is sold is even better, and a product that can taste gourmet, while using poor quality ingredients, is the best of all.

Sanitizing agents are added to keep bacteria from developing in the product, prolonging its shelf life.

Emulsifiers and stabilizers are added to give foods a better texture and homogenous look.

Food coloring is added to create an appealing look.

Flavorings are added to compensate for the bland taste that comes with using substandard ingredients and mass production facilities.

Pesticides and herbicides remain in and on many of the products even after they are processed.

Sweeteners are added to appeal to the sweet tooth in all of us. Many of these sweeteners are far from natural.

Some of these engineered additives have a closer relationship to toxins than they do to nutritional ingredients.

Every time we open a can, box, or packet, every time our children look up at a menu board and tell the clerk their order, we are giving them their daily dose of poison.

How is it that we have come so far from the natural ingredients that our parents fed to us at breakfast lunch and dinner? How is it that we are giving our children foods that can do more harm than good?

The answer is simple: Convenience.

Convenience is that all-powerful time saver. Convenience saves us from spending too much time laboring in the family kitchen. Time better spent driving to work, or in line at the automated teller. How does convenience lead to the existence of dangerous chemicals in our foods?

For the answer we need a history lesson in the art of war.

It all began with Napoleon and his scheme to conquer the world. His troops were scattered all over Europe. Long before the days of transport trucks and refrigeration, nutritional support to his soldiers was a logistical nightmare. One ingenious Frenchman came up with the idea to pour boiling hot soup into wine bottles, cork them, and put them in cases for transport to the front lines. The quality of the soup when it arrived was terrible, and tasted worse, but when you are starving on the front line with a thousand angry soldiers facing you, you enjoyed what little you had.

Thus the idea of packaged lunches began. The bottle may now be a vacuum-sealed plastic tray or tin can, but the nutritional value of the contents has not changed much. What has changed after a few centuries is that technology has allowed us to create additives that mask the blandness of the packaged food, and keep it from spoiling before it reaches our tables.

Early settlers in Canada and United States learned from the French, and began to bottle everything they could. They called this method canning, and each year would store the excess harvest in reusable glass jars. The family farm was a haven for jarred preserves: jams, pickles, beets, corn, and carrots, anything they could gather. The nutritional content of the jarred foods was not as good as fresh, but it was good enough to help keep them fed through the harsh winters.

In the 19th century, as settlers gathered in larger and larger cities, they no longer had the opportunity to farm their own food. Food had to be brought into the cities. Iceboxes were not very large, and few could afford the constant replacement of the ice blocks that had been carved from the lakes and stored from the winter past. More and more value was being placed on packaged foods and perishables.

With the advent of modern mechanization, factories sprang up and became the chief employer in the urban environment. Men who used to come from the fields to dine in the family kitchen would now wait till the whistle blew to open the lunch box that their wives had lovingly filled for them. All too soon the Great War came. Many of the male workforce went off to Europe. The women who had packed their lunches were now packing explosives into bombs, attaching wheels to the field guns and polishing newly forged rifle barrels. These hard working women would come home from the factory floor exhausted, to the hungry faces of their children.

Meals that used to take hours to make needed to take minutes. The day was filled with too many demands to spend hours preparing in the kitchen.

Companies sprang up to come to the aid of mom's hectic schedule. Oscar Mayer, General Foods and Campbell's along with many others heeded the call and started mass producing processed food for the home kitchen.

A whole new industry was born. Convenience foods were here to stay. What they lacked in flavour and nutrition they made up for in ease of preparation. The manufactured food could not compete in flavor or quality with that still made in the family kitchen. To increase their market share, the processed food companies wanted a product that could rival mom's home cooking. They wanted their canned and frozen foods to be so tasty that children would choose their products instead of the home made meal their parents put in front of them. In 1948 the food manufacturers had the answer to their dream. Once again the answer came from war.

In World War II, Japanese soldiers had an advantage over their American counterpart. Their military rations tasted better. This was of great interest to the American military, as well as to the processed food industry. Everyone wanted to know the secret Japanese ingredient that could make substandard grade unpalatable food taste good.

In 1948 representatives from the U.S. Military, Oscar Mayer, General Foods, Campbell's and many other companies in the food industry converged at a symposium in Chicago. The Japanese secret ingredient was unveiled.[24] The ingredient that would make canned and frozen food taste every bit as good as Mom's home made was within reach. The ingredient to make kids crave the food it was added to was now in their grasp. The secret ingredient:

Monosodium Glutamate.

---

[24] Schwartz, Dr. George. In Bad Taste, Health Press, 1999. pg 8.

You've heard the name before. Years ago it was associated with illness after eating in Chinese restaurants. It's not used any more, is it?

Unfortunately Yes. MSG is still a highly used substance added to an enormous number of foods both in restaurants and in prepared grocery items. Almost every restaurant uses it in many of their menu items. It is especially popular as a flavor additive in canned and packaged foods.

Monosodium Glutamate also has a more sinister use:

There are more than 1000 published medical studies that use Monosodium Glutamate. Unlike MSG's use as flavoring in foods, scientific studies use it for two main reasons. Medical researchers appreciate MSG because it gives them consistent, reproducible results every time they use it:

1. When they inject MSG under the skin of newborn mice and rats, it causes the rodents to grow obese beyond their natural range.
2. When they inject MSG directly into a subjects brain cells, it quickly and thoroughly kills them, DEAD.

If Monosodium Glutamate is not a poison, what is?

According to the FDA, MSG is a food additive that can be added to any food in uncontrolled amounts.

Besides making things taste better to people, MSG has some remarkable side-affects including:

Asthma, behavioral problems, stomach cramps, chest discomfort, headache, stomachache, tiredness, depression, nausea, dizziness, loss of bladder/bowel control, rage reactions, and hostility to other children.

Those are just the affects in children. The range of problems MSG causes in adults is twice as large.[25]

If MSG causes dangerous side effects, why would companies all over the U.S. and Canada add it to their products?

MSG has been proven to make foods it is added to more desirable. People will choose a product with the MSG over a similar product that MSG has not been added to.[26]

Other manufacturers, just to keep up with their competition, add MSG to their products, increasing the dosage of it to a higher level then their competitors. The additive war begins, with our children as the casualties.

---

[25] Schwartz, Dr. George. In Bad Taste, Health Press, 1999. pg 53.

[26] Bellisle, F. Dalix, AM. Chapppuis, AS. Rossi, F. Fiquet, P. Gaudin, V. Assoun, M. Slama, G. "Monosodium Glutamate affects mealtime food selection in diabetic patients." **Appetite** 1996 Jun;26(3):267-75.

Monosodium Glutamate: Betcha can't eat just......

So what is this additive and how does it work to make even the blandest foods taste better? More importantly, how is it poisoning my child?

If you go back into your kitchen and look once again at the ingredients lists on the products you find there, you may be shocked to see just what foods list MSG on the label.

Potato Chips	Nachos	Flavored Crackers
Wieners	Bologna	Canned Soup
Canned Pastas	Canned Chili	Ramen Noodles
Vegetable Juice	Dried Soup Mix	Canned Meats
Salad Dressing	Frozen Cured Meats	Frozen Potatoes
Frozen Entrees	Frozen Diet Entrees	Gravy
Seasoning Mix	Cheese puffs	Jerky
Soy Sauce	Ice Cream	Sour Cream
Bouillon Cubes	Pasta Helpers	Flavored Rice

This list is only a small sampling. Chances are, the few items you don't find MSG listed on will have gelatin, autolyzed yeast, yeast extract, hydrolyzed plant or animal protein. These substances contain large amounts of Monosodium Glutamate in their chemical make up. You may even see MSG, hydrolyzed vegetable protein, and autolyzed yeast extract all on the same label. This ensures you get a triple dose in one helping. Meats like frozen chicken breasts often list a percentage of 'meat protein' injected into it. This meat protein is often filled with Glutamate.

Few processed foods are free from the Japanese super ingredient. Even the multi-vitamins you give your children to stay healthy may have MSG hidden in them in the form of gelatin or HVP (hydrolyzed vegetable protein).

Now that you see just how common this substance is in our every day diet, you may want to know just what it is that is going into our mouths.

First patented in 1909, Monosodium Glutamate was produced in Japan and China. By the 1930's, Japan was creating ten million pounds yearly to add to its food supply.

In 1948 it entered the American food chain. Its current popularity in products shows how many companies signed on after the Chicago Symposium.

Almost a hundred years after Monosodium Glutamate received its' first patent, it has been linked to more toxic reactions than almost any other food additive.

Monosodium Glutamate is a form of Amino Acid. Amino acids are the building blocks of proteins found in all living beings. There are 20 types of amino acids used by the human body. Our brain and many major organs in our body use the Glutamate amino acid.

Unlike most chemicals that we eat, MSG passes very quickly into the blood stream and enters the brain and organs directly. Once there, it causes the neurons (nerve endings in the brain and other organs) to fire uncontrollably. The brain translates this over-stimulation of the nerves into what we believe to be good taste and increased flavor. In the stimulated neuron's last few hours of life the neuron fires uncontrollably, sending the excitement of the MSG to our cognitive brain. Two to twenty-four hours later, the neuron is dead, its thought synapses terminated. The mental pathway it had bridged is permanently destroyed. Unfortunately, the brain has difficulty creating new cells, and has to relearn new paths around the damaged area. The brain cells you are born with are designed to last a lifetime. In a few short hours, MSG has excited your brain cells to death.[27]

Have you ever thought that kids today are 'Over stimulated?'

When food tastes better, both children and adults want to eat more of it. In doing so they increase their Glutamate level, causing them to crave more. Is it normal to continue eating after our stomach is no longer interested in food? How often have you opened a bag of snacks, only to look down minutes later to discover you had eaten the whole bag without even realizing it?

Is it any surprise that a record number of children in United States and Canada have been diagnosed with obesity? MSG may well make it easier for them to put on the pounds. In hundreds of studies published in medical journals in North America and abroad, researchers routinely administer Monosodium Glutamate to newborn rats and mice to induce abnormal obesity within days of birth. They then use the affected animals as experimental subjects for research on anything from diabetes to weight loss.

Certainly our governments would protect us from a dangerous chemical, wouldn't they? After all, they thoroughly test all substances to ensure its safety before allowing it into public hands?

No.

At one point, our governments considered both tobacco and asbestos to be safe. Sodium fluoride, a popular rat poison, is considered a safe additive to our water supply.

---

[27] Blaylock, Dr. Russell. Excitotoxins: The Taste that Kills. Health Press, Sante Fe. 1997. Page 42.

Prior to 1958, they were no guidelines in the United States to determine what ingredients could be added to processed foods. In 1958, U.S. Congress established the GRAS list (Generally regarded as safe). They created a list of all known food additives, and sent it out along with a questionnaire to 900 scientists asking them what they thought about the ingredients listed. They reviewed the 355 responses that were returned, and from the written comments approved the list. Of the entire list of additives sent out, only three items were removed, determined dangerous to public health.[28]

Any food additives on the GRAS list can be added to foods with absolutely no limitations.

Despite being listed as an additive generally regarded as safe, the FDA is aware that Glutamate in foods is not as safe as they claim.

The FDA itself in a report dated August 31, 1995, stated that:
Studies have shown that the body uses Glutamate, an amino acid, as a nerve impulse transmitter in the brain and that there are Glutamate-responsive tissues in other parts of the body, as well. Abnormal function of Glutamate receptors has been linked with certain neurological diseases, such as Alzheimer's disease and Huntington's chorea. Injections of Glutamate in laboratory animals have resulted in damage to nerve cells in the brain.

The FDA report went on to say that between 1980 and 1994, there were 622 reports of complaints about side effects from MSG. In 1992, the FDA asked the Federation of American Societies for Experimental Biology to review the available data and make a report about the findings. In the 350 page FASEB report, the Federation concluded that an

"unknown percentage of the population may react to MSG and develop MSG symptom complex, a condition characterized by one or more of the following symptoms:

---

[28] Winter, Ruth. <u>A Consumer's Dictionary of Food Additives.</u> Three Rivers Press, New York, 1999. Page 4.

- *burning sensation in the back of the neck, forearms and chest*

- *numbness in the back of the neck, radiating to the arms and back*

- *tingling, warmth and weakness in the face, temples, upper back, neck and arms*

- *facial pressure or tightness*

- *chest pain*

- *headache*

- *nausea*

- *rapid heartbeat*

- *bronchospasm (difficulty breathing) in MSG-intolerant people with asthma*

- *drowsiness*

- *weakness.*

In otherwise healthy MSG-intolerant people, the MSG symptom complex tends to occur within one hour after eating 3 grams or more of MSG on an empty stomach or without other food. A typical serving of Glutamate-treated food contains less than 0.5 grams of MSG. A reaction is most likely if the MSG is eaten in a large quantity or in a liquid, such as a clear soup."

The FASEB report specified that the above symptoms exist, and manifest themselves in people who are susceptible to MSG. It also states that these symptoms can manifest within an hour of ingesting 3 grams of MSG (about half a teaspoon). Since MSG is a GRAS ingredient, food manufacturers can add as much as they like to any product. Even if the food the report speaks of only has .5 grams, what happens when several MSG ingredients are added? What makes them think that food only has .5 grams of MSG in it?

The report recognizes states that a reaction is more likely if the MSG is eating in soup. Almost all Campbells and Knorr soups contain MSG or ingredients that have glutamate hidden within them.

Considering there are no limits or guidelines set by the FDA, how can the FASEB claim to have any idea how much Glutamate is in any of the foods available on the market?

Michelle and I happen to know from personal experience that we are one of the "unknown percentage" that they speak of. Within minutes of eating anything with MSG, even one serving, the back of the neck becomes very warm and the eyes start to lose focus. Spots of light or colors can be seen hovering in the peripheral vision. The face becomes flushed and hot to the touch, followed quickly by the onset of a headache.

Whatever the percentage of people the FASEB report refers to, be it 10% or 90%, the FDA is not interested in considering any constraints on MSG in food. After receiving this report, the FDA neither asked for more testing to be done nor changed MSG's GRAS status.

The FDA does not seem overly concerned with public safety, as proven by its 1997 decision to change the way a company can get a new additive approved for GRAS standing. It is now a very simple procedure for a manufacturer to put a new ingredient into a product. Manufacturers need only send a letter of notification to the FDA declaring that their additive is generally regarded as safe, and attach a couple of scientific studies that they themselves have done. Faster than you can say 'rubber stamp', the FDA approves it and the manufacturer is free to add as much of the new ingredient to your food as they want.

Without any help from the FDA, we are forced to do our own research into the safety of food additives.

When I was studying at university, a talented psychology professor took me on as a research assistant. I learned how to search through journal articles, decipher abstracts, even coordinate, run and analyze experiments. Many great studies are done every year, each with a little piece of the puzzle that could one day unlock the answers we seek. Unfortunately the vast majority of these studies are never heard of, buried in scientific jargon and hidden away in dusty barely visited corridors. It was in these publications that I found the answer: Hundreds of studies showing the dangers of MSG. I was shocked that the FDA had not banned MSG long ago.

There are side effects of MSG that were not even mentioned in the FASEB report.

From obesity and diabetes to Alzheimer's and autism, studies show a mountain of undeniable evidence that eating Monosodium Glutamate can do long term, irreversible damage to the body.

MSG, a Moment on the Lips, forever in your......

Glutamate is one of the most powerful chemicals in the body. It is the main neurotransmitter used in the brain. Glutamate affects almost every organ in the body. Eating Monosodium Glutamate upsets the natural balance of glutamate in the body, and it does so with profound and long lasting effects.

The following are twelve of the serious diseases and afflictions that scientific evidence has linked to glutamate. With further research, who knows how many more side effects will come to light.

Monosodium Glutamate and Obesity

With a greater frequency, Canadian and American children are becoming 'obese'. Obesity in adults and children is at its record high. According to the 1999-2000 U.S. National Health and Nutrition Examination Survey (NHANES) 15 percent of children and adolescents ages 6-19 years are overweight. This is a large increase from the 11 percent found in a similar survey done in 1984. It was an even larger jump from the 5% obesity rates found from 1970 to 1960. In Canada the number of obese children rose from 5 to 13.5% between the years of 1981 and 1996.[29]

Even among adults, obesity rates are on the rise. The prevalence of obesity among US adults climbed from 19.8 percent to 20.9 percent between 2000 and 2001. 44.3 million U.S. residents (1 in every 5) were found to be obese. In Canada 1 in 6 adults is obese, while 50% of the entire adult population is considered overweight.

These trends in unhealthy body weight are costly to the community as a whole, as well as to the individual. In the U.S., illnesses linked to being overweight cost $100 billion in medical expenses and lost productivity. The cost in human life is even greater. Half a million people die every year of illnesses directly related to obesity.

In today's world, the easiest thing to do is to consume. We tend to have everything delivered and we eat every meal as if it were our last.

Lethargy is setting in. Hundreds of channels on T.V. to watch, thousands of video games to play, fast paced stressful lives filled with mega-huge combo platters with 2000 calories in one meal.

With both parents working, and no time to cook meals from scratch, convenience has become the name of the game. We are seduced daily with the draw of fast food establishments. In 1970, Americans were spending $6 billion on fast food. In 2000, the fast food market leapt to $110 billion.[30]

Everyday we are influenced by advertising that brain washes our children into begging us to 'go here, eat there.' Even in schools one cannot escape the fast food chains. Pizza Hut, Taco Bell, Coke, Pepsi, and many more multinational corporations are paying the school boards to have their food and drink exclusively served in the cafeterias. Snacks and convenience foods are the order of the new millennium. 'Mom, Dad, let's go to that restaurant, they make better chicken then you do.' How can parents argue? mom and dad

---

[29] Tremblay MS, Willms JD. "Secular trends in the body mass index of Canadian children." CMAJ 2000;163:1429-33.

[30] Sclosser, Eric. Fast Food Nation, Houghton Mifflin, 2001. Page 3.

just can't compete with the convenience, fast delivery, and taste. It's simply because they don't know the secret ingredient that makes even the cheapest cuts of meat and blandest of vegetables burst with flavour. Mom and dad forgot to add MSG to their meatloaf! No wonder they can't compete. Just a sprinkle of MSG can make a quick meal taste like a carefully prepared banquet. The taste alone makes you want to eat until everything's gone.

The end result is a western population that is more overweight than any other population on the planet.

Parents and doctors are scrambling to point to a specific culprit. Perhaps it is laziness, high caloric intake, poor diet, or genetics.

All of these factors can be part of the problem, but MSG can be the link to all of them. Not only can exposure to MSG predispose children to obesity, but it may also reduce their activity level and hamper their ability to shed excess weight. Children given large amounts of MSG may gain weight even though they eat less than other children. Genetics too may be a problem. If a developing fetus is exposed to high levels of MSG in the mothers diet, it could make the infant more prone to weight gain later in life.

Hundreds of studies have been made using MSG in laboratory experiments. Though manufacturers of MSG proclaim its safety independent laboratory experiments have not proven it. The world's population has become the biggest experimental test pool of all. By letting toxins like MSG into our food supply, we are seeing the results on a global scale.

Independent researchers appreciate the amazing consistently reproducible powers of Monosodium Glutamate. They have seen it in mice and rats; we can see it when we look in the mirror.

In a study of mice given doses of MSG shortly after birth, it was discovered that the entire group of mice became obese. Fat tissue mass was 65% more than the control group that did not get any MSG.[31] Hundreds of studies have produced the same result:

---

[31] Moss, D. Ma, A. Cameron, DP. "Defective thermoregulatory thermogenesis in Monosodium Glutamate-induced obesity in mice." **Metabolism** 1985 Jul;34(7):626-30.

guaranteed obesity. Researchers who want to test a new diet drug inject newborn mice or rats with MSG, and presto, in a matter of weeks you have morbidly obese mice. Ready for any diet drug or chemical you want to throw their way. This group of experimental mice even has a name: "MSG-treated mice." Not very imaginative, but when you mention the term in the right academic circles, people in lab coats are likely to give a knowing nod.

Another repetitive feature of "MSG-treated mice" is hyperinsulinemia, a condition where the pancreas excretes huge amounts of insulin. Increased insulin stores away the glucose in the blood by converting it to the adipose tissue we know as fat. The increased insulin is what creates the obese response in the mice and rats.[32] Hyperinsulinemia is directly linked to the development of diabetes.

One of the main reasons that mice and rats are tested with experimental drugs meant for humans, is that out of all the animal kingdom, their physiology closely mimics ours.

If Monosodium Glutamate affects rodents in this way, what could it do to humans?

Like the MSG-Treated Mice, our weight and insulin level are also be affected by extra Glutamates in our blood stream.

The FDA report dated August 31, 1995 pointed out *"there are Glutamate-responsive tissues in other parts of the body."* They did not go into more detail, but one of those Glutamate-responsive tissues is the pancreas. The pancreas is designed to recognize when blood sugar levels are too high and sends out insulin to change the sugar into fat tissue to be stored.

The amino acid, Glutamate, tells the pancreas when and how much insulin to create. Insulin determines just how much fat you will

---

[32] Cameron, DP. Cutbush, L. Opat, F. "Effects of Monosodium Glutamate-induced obesity in mice on carbohydrate metabolism in insulin secretion." **Clin Exp Pharmacol Physiol** 1978 Jan-Feb;5(1):41-51.

store on your body. An over efficient pancreas can cause a great deal of fat deposits to develop on the body.When abnormally high levels of Glutamate are introduced to the insulin-making beta cells of the pancreas, these mini-factories switch into overdrive. They create massive amounts of insulin that pours into the blood stream. The levels of insulin the cells produce are directly related to how much Glutamate is stimulating them.[33] This finding would help explain the connection to weight gain. Monosodium Glutamate enters into the blood stream from the food we eat. It winds its way through the entire body, finding Glutamate receptors in many of the major organs.

Even if all you had was a salad and low-calorie, low-fat dressing, the insulin still rushes out. There might be next to no blood sugar in your veins, but the MSG that can be found in the salad dressing has tickled your pancreas, unleashing a torrent of fat-creating insulin. The insulin wanders around your body like an army, finding any sugars it can to turn into adipose tissue and store it away in areas we commonly refer to as love handles or thunder thighs.

If you or someone you know has a history of weight issues, you could be one of 'those' that the FDA refers to as being susceptible to MSG. Your weight problem may have a direct correlation with the ingestion of MSG.

The battle of the bulge begins:

It's Saturday just after lunch and you're proud of yourself for sticking to your diet and avoiding the french fries and apple pie that your kids got at the drive-through. Back at home, the kids play computer games family room and it's time to do those 20 minutes of exercising that you promised yourself you'd do. But wait, where did that urge to workout go? All you had was a salad with low-cal dressing and your body is so drained that it is ready for a nap. What happened to the motivation? The smiling girl on the

---

[33] Hoy, M. Maechler, P. Efanov, AM. Wollheim, CB. Berggren, PO. Gromada, J. "Increase in cellular Glutamate levels stimulates exocytosis in pancreatic beta-cells." **FEBS Lett** 2002 Nov 6;531(2):199-203.

workout tape can't even inspire it in you. 'Maybe if I just lay down, that's it, maybe a little nap would help.......zzzzzzzzz.....'

'Ahhh, that was a relaxing nap. Now I can work out. Hmmm, I am a little hungry'. The insulin in your blood has stripped your body of all excess sugar, leaving you hypoglycemic and yearning for something sweet. 'No, I can't have sweets; it'll blow my diet. I'll just have a couple low fat vegetable crackers, that should do me.' The first cracker hits your tongue. You savor it, making it last. 'Boy, these crackers sure taste extra good!' The Monosodium Glutamate in the crackers enters your blood almost instantly. It makes a beeline to your brain where it tells you that these are the tastiest crackers ever; just a few more won't hurt.

You sit down on the couch. You've turned off the fitness tape, and now the television comes on. 'That was a good show, is an hour up already?' You look down and see that you've eaten the whole box of vegetable crackers. 'Yikes, how did that happen? I didn't know I was that hungry.' Well, I can make up for the extra calories by not having supper. I am sure to lose weight that way!' So you grit your teeth and try to resist the dinner you make for your family. You really don't want to spend a lot of time in that tempting kitchen, so you toss some frozen low fat chicken teriyaki and rice in the oven. Meanwhile, the MSG from the crackers is surging through you, seeking out the pancreas once again. Once more insulin pours out, this time finding carbohydrates to grab onto and stuff on your abdomen or thighs. You had a nap, but still can't figure out why you feel so drained.

'I'll go to bed early tonight, that will help', you say to yourself as you dish out the steaming portions to your family. You pour the vegetable juice. You smile, glad that they are eating healthy. The precooked stir-fry looks good, and smells great. You can't believe its low in fat! Unfortunately for you it isn't low in MSG.

Fat molecules carry much of the flavor in food. When manufacturers of diet food take out the fat, they have to put in flavor somehow. So they pile on the MSG. Thanks to the FDA, there are no limits to how much Glutamate they add. Sure enough, the low fat chicken teriyaki with rice could list as ingredients Monosodium Glutamate, hydrolyzed plant protein, autolyzed yeast extract, soy sauce, maybe even gelatin and sodium caseinate. Unwittingly, you may have just served your family seven servings of Glutamates in one meal, and the package called itself 'healthy'!

So now your spouse and childrens are on the same roller coaster you've been riding. They've been on it since breakfast, the sausages and hash browns, the chicken or hamburger at the fast food restaurant. Their blood is packed with even more insulin. Loads of carbohydrates have arrived for it to feast on, especially the low fat cheesecake they just had for dessert. You wonder why your kids are getting a little plump. Why don't they want to go outside? When you were a kid, you couldn't wait to get outside on a beautiful sunny day. All they want to do is play video games or watch 150 channels of T.V.

The reality is, they are just as robbed of motivation as you were today.

The culprit: Monosodium Glutamate, possibly the secret ingredient for the ultimate Yo-Yo diet.

But the insult is yet to come. On Sunday morning you step on the scale, smiling with pride at yesterday's resolve: salad and a few crackers. But wait! The smile leaves your face. 'This thing must be broken! How could it be?' The scale isn't lying; you've gained a pound! You head for the kitchen, more starved than ever, choking back your frustration. The fudge brownie walnut ice cream is beckoning. 'If I'm gonna gain a pound, I might as well enjoy it!'

You look at your kids and hope they outgrow the weight issues they have even now. 'They're young, they'll grow into their weight.' As long as MSG drains their physical motivation, they are unlikely to become the energized children you are hoping to see. As long as your children have MSG in their diet, it may continue to work against them and could damn them to a life of obesity and lethargy.

Any individuals who are sensitive to MSG (that undetermined percentage of the population that the FDA identifies) and try to diet to lose the weight, could have any or even all of the following factors working against them.

> ➤ The Glutamate present in MSG and other artificial food additives over- stimulates the pancreas creating large amounts of insulin even when only a small amount of food is eaten. Cameron, Cutbush and Opat in a study done as far back as 1978 determined that mice who receive doses of MSG shortly after birth became obese, even though "after weaning, food intake in MSG-treated mice is less than control mice."[34] They also determined that after the fast that naturally occurs at night, MSG treated mice were hyperglycemic, having significantly less blood sugar than their non-MSG counterparts.[35] Even while they slept, their pancreases excreted enough insulin to store away what little sugar they had left in their blood, expediently turning it into fat. Do you know anyone who 'eats like a bird' but is still on the heavy side?

> ➤ The motivation to exercise is almost impossible to find. The hyperinsulinemia that MSG can trigger sends large amounts of insulin out to sop up almost all the blood sugar it can find.[36] Low blood sugar leaves people feeling drained and exhausted, not at all inspired to hit the jogging trail or head to the gym for aerobics.

> ➤ Experimental test subjects injected with MSG shortly after birth showed a significant reduction in energy activity

---

[34] Cameron, DP. Cutbush, L. Opat, F. "Effects of Monosodium Glutamate-induced obesity in mice on carbohydrate metabolism in insulin secretion." **Clin Exp Pharmacol Physiol** 1978 Jan-Feb;5(1):41-51.

[35] Cameron, DP. Cutbush, L. Opat, F. "Effects of Monosodium Glutamate-induced obesity in mice on carbohydrate metabolism in insulin secretion." **Clin Exp Pharmacol Physiol** 1978 Jan-Feb;5(1):41-51.

[36] Cameron, DP. Cutbush, L. Opat, F. "Effects of Monosodium Glutamate-induced obesity in mice on carbohydrate metabolism in insulin secretion." **Clin Exp Pharmacol Physiol** 1978 Jan-Feb;5(1):41-51.

level.[37]   This discovery could change the way we think about people with obesity. Next time you see a heavy set person on the street, or maybe even in the mirror, consider that their/your situation could be due to MSG triggered lethargy, not the laziness some people may accuse them/you of.

➢ Females that are reactive to MSG may have more weight to lose than males. In a laboratory study between an MSG treated group of males and females, the males, though exhibiting obesity, did not become as obese as the females.[38]

➢ The same study also showed that MSG lowered the amount of growth hormones present during the developmental stage of both female and male subjects. The effect of this was greater in males, who were considerably smaller than their male control counterparts. MSG not only makes one fatter, but shorter as well.

You may be one of the lucky ones. For you weight loss might just mean cutting all free Glutamate out of your diet, thus increasing your energy level and ability to exercise.

For many people, it's not that easy, they may have the worst factor of all: Genetics. Not the genetics caused by inheritance from your parents, but genetics caused by chemicals altering your genes when you are being formed in the womb.

In April of 2003, Oken & Gillman, of the Department of Nutrition, Harvard School of Public Health, published a review of the 'Fetal Origins of Obesity." In their study they reviewed a great deal of studies. This extensive review prompted them to consider the possibility that tendency for weight problems can be determined

---

[37] Poon, TK. Cameron, DP. "Measurement of oxygen consumption and locomotor activity in Monosodium Glutamate-induced obesity." **Am J Physiol** 1978 May;234(5):E532-4.

[38] Maiter, D. Underwood, LE. Martin, JB. Koenig, JI. "Neonatal treatment with Monosodium Glutamate: effects of prolonged growth hormone (GH)-releasing hormone deficiency on pulsatile GH secretion and growth in female rats." Endocrinology 1991 Feb;128(2):1100-6

when a person is still in the womb. They surmised that children had a higher chance of becoming obese if they had the following traits:

1. Low birth weight.
2. Higher than normal mechanisms that increased fat tissue.
3. Abnormal insulin secretion.

These discoveries confounded them.[39] How could low birth weight babies become obese adults? What could manipulate all these factors while the baby was still forming?

These researchers were missing the magic ingredient: Monosodium Glutamate. MSG could solve their riddle for them.

Neonatal mice treated with MSG :

1. Show a deficiency in growth hormone which causes them to grow slower than other mice.[40]
2. Have enlarged adipose tissues (fat storage cells).[41]
3. Have extremely high levels of insulin secretion.[42]

Repeatable, reliable, MSG side effects may be the developmental cause of obesity that Oken & Gillman were looking for.

MSG has been proven to directly affect the unborn fetus. In a 1984 study by Frieder & Grimm, pregnant rats were given water laced with MSG during their second and third trimester. The study discovered that these babies were born with juvenile obesity, reduced energy level, and specific learning disabilities. The study

---

[39] Oken, E. Gillman, MW. "Fetal origins of obesity." **Obes Res** 2003 Apr;11(4):496-506.

[40] Maiter, D. Underwood, LE. Martin, JB. Koenig, JI. "Neonatal treatment with Monosodium Glutamate: effects of prolonged growth hormone (GH)-releasing hormone deficiency on pulsatile GH secretion and growth in female rats." **Endocrinology** 1991 Feb;128(2):1100-6.

[41] Oida, K. Nakai, T. Hayashi, T. Miyabo, S. Takeda, R. "Plasma lipoproteins of Monosodium Glutamate-induced obese rats." **Int J Obes** 1984;8(5):385-91.

[42] Cameron, DP. Cutbush, L. Opat, F. "Effects of Monosodium Glutamate-induced obesity in mice on carbohydrate metabolism in insulin secretion." **Clin Exp Pharmacol Physiol** 1978 Jan-Feb;5(1):41-51.

also proved that MSG crosses the placental barrier, and enters the developing fetus from the mother's blood.[43]

With studies like these illustrating the link between MSG and overactive insulin creation, obesity, and lethargy, it becomes obvious why there could be more and more obese people in America having a difficult time losing weight.

You have heard the stories on the talk shows and news reports. Some people claim that they try everything but can't lose weight. These people may resort to severe surgery such as stomach stapling to help them win the war against unhealthy fat.

The majority of people who suffer from extreme obesity (which doctors refer to as morbid obesity) are female. Males rarely show the potential for extreme obesity that females do. This fact is also reproduced in laboratory studies with rodents. Female subjects respond to MSG induced obesity in a far more extreme way than male counterparts.

Many doctors still believe that the cause of obesity is all in the heads of those afflicted; that extremely obese people have no excuse for being this fat. These doctors would do well to examine the studies that prove that MSG in the mother's diet directly affects the developing fetus. These dramatically obese people may be cursed from birth. Perhaps the obese people are right and the doctors are wrong, maybe it really isn't their entire fault.

For those of you just fighting a few extra pounds, reducing Glutamate intake may be enough to get you back on the road to recovery. Without MSG in your system, your pancreas may return to normal insulin production levels. Without the extra insulin in your body, your blood sugar level will rise to give you a higher energy level. The higher energy level will make it easier for you to get motivated and exercise. Your journey to the ideal weight may not be a long one after all.

---

[43] Frieder, B. Grimm, VE. "Prenatal Monosodium Glutamate (MSG) treatment given through the mother's diet causes behavioral deficits in rat offspring." **Int J Neurosci** 1984 Apr;23(2):117-26.

For those of you who may be obese due to genetics caused by the amount of MSG your mother ate while you were forming in the womb. Your road may be far more difficult. Cutting Glutamate from your diet would only be the first step. There is hope.

When a poison is finally identified, the antidote is easier to find.

Diabetes and MSG, The Hidden Link?

My cousin Jonathon was a fun-loving child. His house was the most fabulous place to visit. He always knew just how to have a good time. His father, a doctor, had passed away when he was young. His mother worked hard to give him the best of everything: stylish clothes, the latest toys, and the tastiest foods. She always gave him the best pre-packaged meals money could buy. Snacks anytime he wanted. I especially enjoyed sleepovers at his house, one in particular.

It was shortly after my Grandmother died. She had been diagnosed with diabetes and had to move from the farm and leave my Grandpa there alone. I was a regular visitor at her retirement home. She always hugged me with a smile, and I always hugged her and smiled back. Then the diabetes got worse, and she was sent off to the extended care unit of the hospital. She still hugged me with a smile, but it was harder for me to smile back. One of her legs had been amputated. 'Diabetes does that' the doctor said. The next time I went, she smiled at me from her wheel chair. Her other leg was now gone. Though her hug was filled with love, it was very hard for me to smile that time. I was sorry that I didn't smile. The next time I saw her was at the funeral home.

My parents knew a stay at Jonathon's house would cheer me up. So they packed me up and dropped me off.

Sure enough, by 1:00 am, surrounded by potato chips, nachos, the most decadent cookies and candies, we were kicking back watching late night TV. He always was the best at telling a joke and we spent as much time laughing as we did gorging ourselves. I cringed when he made a prank phone call, but deep down I thought he was the coolest and bravest kid I knew, a real hero. For the moment, I forgot my Grandma, the diabetes, the missing smile. At 13 it's easy to find joyful diversions.

I was sure Jonathon had the best life: falling to sleep to the Letterman show, eating at fast food places more than at home. Wow, if only I had it so good. I envied all he had going for him. Until he turned 18 and it all came crashing down.

Diabetes killed my Grandmother, and now it took hold of my cousin. At age 18 he was diagnosed with juvenile diabetes, and would need daily insulin injections for the rest of his life. I was scared to see him after that. I was even afraid to call him on the phone. I haven't seen him since those teenage years. It's sad really, cause he truly deserves a smile.

I ask my father what Jonathon's doing now. He dealt with the needles, the lifestyle change, the pain, and the fear. He overcame it all to graduate with honors in biology. Right now he is working with a team of scientists to find new ways to save people's lives. He is still my hero, after all.

It's memories like this that keep us all going. So with thoughts of loved ones on my mind, I strove to research as much as I could into what had caused hardship to those around me.

Just what is diabetes?

Diabetes occurs when the pancreas fails to produce enough insulin to regulate the sugar levels in the blood. How could the pancreas fail?

We have already seen that high doses of Monosodium Glutamate in growing mice and rats produce hyperinsulinemia, the condition where the pancreas dramatically increases the amount of insulin in the blood. Consider for a moment what happens when an organ becomes over-worked. The liver, kidneys, and heart are all susceptible to failure when they are constantly stressed. A heart racing continually at 200 beats a minute for more than a few days could certainly bring on heart failure.

Imagine a pancreas, pumping out 50-100 percent more than the usual amount of insulin. For a while, years perhaps, the pancreas continues to function, but at some point, the stress can be too much. The pancreas fails and the result is the harsh reality: Diabetes.

Diabetes affects 17 million Americans, and over 2 million Canadians. The number of cases grows more rapidly every year. The American Diabetes Association reports that there are 16 million more Americans with pre-diabetes, a condition where the pancreas is not producing enough insulin to regulate blood levels, but not at serious enough levels to be diagnosed. That's a total of 33 million Americans whose pancreases are failing to do their job.

According to these figures, more than one in ten people in the United States have pancreases that have either started to or completely lost the ability to perform. Diabetes has been around for thousands of years, but only in this century has it grown to epidemic proportions. In the U.S. alone, one million people aged 20 and over are diagnosed with diabetes every year.

At this rate, 1 in 4 people in the U.S. could have diabetes by 2053. Look at your family, your children, your grandchildren. Who will it be?

Diabetes is the number one cause of death by disease in North America. It is the leading cause of blindness; it increases the chance of heart disease 2 to 4 times; it accounts for a quarter of all new cases of kidney disease; it is the reason for 50% of limb amputations around the world. Chances are, you or your children could get it at some point in life. It is a difficult, all-encompassing disease. As parents we need to worry most because juvenile diabetes (Type 1) is the most debilitating. As the name suggests, its number one victim is children.

What causes diabetes?

Both the American and the Canadian Diabetes Associations have no answer. Some would point to the increase in sugar consumption. Larger and larger amounts of refined sugar in the western diet may exacerbate diabetes. But according to the Canadian Diabetes Association, eating too much sugar does not cause it.

Monosodium Glutamate can.

Glutamate is the main excitatory neurotransmitter in mammals.[44] It affects the operation of almost every organ. Nerves that are excited by Glutamate are found in the heart, nervous system, kidney, liver, lung, spleen, and testis.[45] The pancreas is the organ responsible for the regulation of all sugar (glucose) levels in the blood. When sugar levels in the blood are too high signals are sent to the Beta-cells within the pancreas telling them to create insulin. Monosodium Glutamate in the blood stream can bypass the regular control of the pancreas and hyper stimulate the beta- cells to over-produce insulin.[46]

In the previous chapter on obesity, it was shown how injection of MSG into newborn rats leads to hyperinsulinemia. Hyperinsulinemia is the process of Glutamate's hyper stimulation of the pancreas that causes overproduction of insulin, leading to obesity. Hyperinsulinemia facilitates fuel storage as fat.[47] It can be the first step to diabetes.

---

[44] Monfort, P. Munoz, MD. ElAyadi, A. Kosenko, E., Felipo, V. "Effects of hyperammonemia and liver failure on Glutamatergic neurotransmission." **Metab Brain Dis** 2002 Dec;17(4):237-50.

[45] Gill, SS. Mueller, RW. McGuire, PF. Pulido, OM. "Potential target sites in peripheral tissues for excitatory neurotransmission and excitotoxicity." **Toxicol Pathol** 2000 Mar-Apr;28(2):277-84.

[46] Hoy, M. Maechler, P. Efanov, AM. Wollheim, CB. Berggren,PO. Gromada, J. "Increase in cellular Glutamate levels stimulates exocytosis in pancreatic beta-cells." **FEBS Lett** 2002 Nov 6;531(2):199-203.

[47] Girod, JP. Brotman, DJ. "The metabolic syndrome as a vicious cycle: does obesity beget obesity?" **Med Hypotheses** 2003 Apr;60(4):584-9.

Obese and overweight people have the greatest likelihood of developing diabetes in their lifetime. With the evidence gathered from studies, a new question is brought to light. Do people develop diabetes because they are overweight, or does the same thing cause both their obesity and subsequent diabetes: Monosodium Glutamate?

Consider the following situation:

Sally has been attending school for years, following the same routine. She eats the school lunch (high in MSG), sits in a class all day, and returns home to snack on more MSG laden foods. As we have seen in studies, MSG stimulates the pancreas to create extra insulin that in turn lowers the blood sugar leading to lethargy that her parents label as 'laziness'. She ends up watching T.V, having little energy for anything else. Sally finds it difficult to get motivated to exercise, even though she promises herself she will try. MSG has her sinking into a deeper trap.

Over the years, the weight piles on. She doesn't even eat as much as her friends and still she gains weight. Soon she is part of the growing population of obese children in America. Her pancreas, continually overexcited by the MSG she has eaten literally every day, is starting to shut down. The beta cells are deteriorating and the body's T-cell immune system comes in to shut them down. Her pancreas fails a little more each day. By the time she is in her twenties, she is on the verge of Type 2 diabetes. Her pancreas can no longer produce enough insulin for the requirements that her brain has requested. Soon the pills prescribed by the doctor become daily injections.

How did she get to this point? Sally is not alone in her life sentence. There are millions out there just like her.

They sit in silence, judged and condemned by those who are healthier. They try a thousand ways to diet, but whatever they manage to lose comes back with a vengeance.

They hear the constant criticism: 'Heavy people are just lazy.' 'They overeat, they do it to themselves.'

Even in this enlightened age, professionals fall into the simple trap of blaming the victim.

In a recent study by Dr. Frank B. Hu and colleagues at the Harvard School of Public Health and Brigham and Women's Hospital, the routines of 50,000 nurses were studied. During the six years of this study, 3,750 of these women became obese, and 1,515 developed diabetes. Dr. Frank Hu pointed to the two hours of daily TV watching as the culprit, along with the eating of high-calorie, fat-rich foods. Almost half of the women who became obese developed diabetes. His answer to this problem: get up and walk around for two hours.[48] Easy for him to say, but impossible for them to do.

It is likely that MSG was in their blood, lowering their blood sugar levels to near drowsiness and causing them to yearn for more food. Then the MSG stimulated the pancreas to death, leaving a life sentence of diabetes.

There can be yet one more factor to exacerbate the problem of both diabetes and morbid obesity. In extreme cases of both, the victims tend to be hospitalized or institutionalized in retirement homes. While in these facilities their sugar intake is controlled, but not their MSG intake. Institutions tend to use a great deal of MSG to make their mass-produced meals more palatable. The MSG may be counteracting all the good these places could do for their diabetic patients.

It may not be too late for us. The studies are there for us to learn from. The over-stimulation of the pancreas is directly related to the MSG that we ingest.[49] [50]

---

[48] Edelson, Ed. "Watching too much television is dangerous for your body." **HealthScoutNews** April 8, 2003.

[49] Graham, TE. Sgro, V. Friars, D. Gibala, MJ. "Glutamate ingestion: the plasma and muscle free amino acid pools of resting humans." **Am J Physiol Endocrinol Metab** 2000 Jan;278(1):E83-9.

[50] Mourtzakis, M. Graham, TE. "Glutamate ingestion and its effects at rest and during exercise in humans." **J Appl Physiol** 2002 Oct;93(4):1251-9.

This may well be the simplest cure for Diabetes:

1. If we do not eat MSG, our pancreases will not be over stimulated.

2. If the pancreas is not producing too much insulin, we will not become obese and lethargic.

3. If we do not become obese and become lethargic, we will be less likely to get diabetes.

4. The end result is a healthier population.

Losing weight could be as simple as cutting MSG from the diet. The population of the western world is becoming obese at an alarming rate. We now have the power to stop it.

Glutamate and Eye Health.

The human eye is extremely sensitive to changes in Glutamate levels. The capillaries in the eye easily transport glutamate directly into the sensitive areas of the eye. This is especially apparent when Monosodium Glutamate is ingested. Subjects fed on a high diet of MSG developed retinas with extremely thin membranes. Researchers found that a diet of MSG over several years could result in retinal cell destruction and total blindness.[51]

Diabetes is the leading cause of blindness in United States and Canada. For years, diabetes research has focused on Retinopathy, or enlarging of the blood vessels in the eye, as the cause of blindness in people diagnosed with diabetes. New studies suggest that retinopathy is not the cause of blindness, but rather the catalyst by which the cells within the retina are destroyed. When the blood vessels become enlarged due to high blood sugar, the spaces between the cell membranes also enlarge. This allows for the

---

[51] Ohguro, H. Katsushima, H. Maruyama, I. Maeda, T. Yanagihashi, S. Metoki, T. Nakazawa, M. "A high dietary intake of sodium Glutamate as flavoring (ajinomoto) causes gross changes in retinal morphology and function." **Exp Eye Res** 2002 Sep;75(3):307-15.

already thin membrane to become very permeable to the Glutamate. Glutamate in the blood passes directly into the structures of the eye.[52] Glutamate in the eye seeks out the glial cells which support vision, latching onto them and exciting them to death.[53]

Glaucoma, another condition found often in diabetics, is a result of dead cells accumulating within the eye. As research shows, few chemicals in the body are as efficient at killing nerve cells than Glutamate. By ingesting large amounts of MSG in their diet, diabetics could be greatly increasing their chances of going blind.

It is not only those with diabetes that need to be concerned about their vision. We should be concerned for our growing children as well.

Monosodium Glutamate can damage the eyes in rats as they grow. MSG given to newborn rats caused disturbances of eyeball growth. The layers of the retina began to degenerate causing the rat to develop vision problems.[54]

Our children's eyes are not fully formed at birth and continue to develop into adolescence. Could Glutamate have a degenerated affect on our children? The Glutamate Association, an organization that promotes and champions the use of MSG in all food products, claims that MSG is safe for babies as well as adults. Twenty years ago, however, food manufacturers voluntarily removed MSG from baby food and infant formula. Did their researchers discover something that they are not telling us? Has there been an increase in children needing glasses earlier in life, and could it be due to MSG in the diet?

Further research into this area is definitely needed.

---

[52] Antonetti, DA. Lieth, E. Barber, AJ. Gardner, TW. "Molecular mechanisms of vascular permeability in diabetic retinopathy." **Semin Ophthalmol** 1999 Dec;14(4):240-8.

[53] Barber, AJ. "A new view of diabetic retinopathy: a neurodegenerative disease of the eye." **Prog Neuropsychopharmacol Biol Psychiatry** 2003 Apr;27(2):283-90.

[54] Kawamura, M. Azuma, N. Kohsaka, S. "Experimental studies on microphthalmos formation in neonatal rats treated with monosodium-L-Glutamate." Nippon Ganka Gakkai Zasshi 1989 May;93(5):553-61.

Blood Brain Barrier: Invasion of the Glutamate

A careful balance of amino acids runs the human body. When these elements become over-represented in the body, chaos can ensue. The FDA claims that MSG cannot cross the blood brain barrier, though the studies to support this are sparse. This is not surprising considering the level of neural-knowledge available in 1948 when MSG was first introduced to America. We should not forget the complete lack of research done when the FDA introduced the GRAS list in 1958 that declared MSG to be safe in any quantity.

Glutamate is not only one of the most important neurotransmitters in the brain, it is also recognized by scientists to be an excitotoxin. Excitotoxins in the brain can result in massive cell death.[55]

If excess Glutamate were to cross the blood brain barrier, neurons within the brain would be in great jeopardy.

The FDA clings to the mistaken belief that MSG cannot cross the blood brain barrier. If Glutamate could pass the BBB, it would no longer be considered a harmless ingredient and be able to be added in unlimited amounts to your food. Glutamate is an excitotoxin

---

[55] Singh, P. Mann, KA. Mangat, HK. Kaur, G. "Prolonged Glutamate excitotoxicity: effects on mitochondrial antioxidants and antioxidant enzymes." **Mol Cell Biochem** 2003 Jan;243(1-2):139-45.

capable of killing the cells of the brain.[56] What the FDA has overlooked is the fact that the blood brain barrier is not infallible, and can fail in many situations.

Increased physical stress of a short duration can increase the ease with which larger molecules can cross into the brain.[57] Brain injury (stroke or trauma), where a blood vessel breaks and bleeds into the brain, allows direct access for the MSG to cross the barrier and enter the brain.[58]

Allergies create an increase in histamine in the blood. Histamine dilates the arterioles, allowing for larger molecules to enter the brain.[59]

The brain is not completely protected. The hypothalamus is an important organ that regulates hormones throughout the body. It is linked to growth and the control of the pituitary gland. The Hypothalamus does not benefit from having a blood barrier, and can be directly influenced by MSG in the blood stream.[60] The lack of protection from Glutamates can allow MSG to impair memory retention and damage neurons in the hypothalamus.[61]

Another region that the FDA seems to have completely forgot about is the meninges. This is the lining between your brain and your skull. It is filled with tiny capillaries, which researchers are now finding have transporter cells dedicated to the transport of Glutamate into the brain.

---

[56] Dodd, PR. "Excited to death: different ways to lose your neurons." **Biogerontology** 2002;3(1-2):51-6.

[57] Skultetyova, I. Tokarev, D. Jezova, D. "Stress-induced increase in blood-brain barrier permeability in control and Monosodium Glutamate-treated rats." **Brain Res Bull** 1998;45(2):175-8.

[58] Gilgun-Sherki, Y. Rosenbaum, Z. Melamed, E. Offen, D. "Antioxidant therapy in acute central nervous system injury: current state." **Pharmacol Rev** 2002 Jun;54(2):271-84.

[59] Mayhan, WG. "Role of nitric oxide in histamine-induced increases in permeability of the blood-brain barrier." **Brain Res** 1996 Dec 16;743(1-2):70-6.

[60] Blaylock, Dr. Russell. "Excitotoxins: The Taste that Kills." Health Press, 1997. Page 19.

[61] Park, CH. Choi, SH. Piao, Y. Kim, S. Lee, YJ. Kim, HS. Jeong, SJ. Rah, JC. Seo, JH. Lee, JH. Chang, K. Jung, YJ. Suh, YH. "Glutamate and aspartate impair memory retention and damage hypothalamic neurons in adult mice." **Toxicol Lett** 2000 May 19;115(2):117-25.

The Ajinomoto Company on its own corporate Website clearly outlines another way that MSG can directly enter the brain. In a page designed to sell its Glutamate to research laboratories, Ajinomoto states that L-Glutamate (MSG) and ammonia combine to form L-Glutamine Acid. Ajinomoto Company states that L-Glutamine can pass through the blood brain barrier. L-Glutamine can break down into Glutamate and Ammonia.[62] This can directly increase the neurotoxic levels of Glutamate in the brain.

The FDA has blindly stated that MSG cannot cross the blood brain barrier where it could endanger the sensitive brain processes. MSG's manufacturer promotes the fact that it can. What has happened here? This kind of contradiction is even worse than the tobacco companies knowing that nicotine was addictive and still advocating its safety. Ajinomoto directly promotes the effects MSG can have on the brain, and the FDA turns a blind eye to it.

The bottom line is that Monosodium Glutamate in the diet can enter the brain. The question is, once it is there, what evils can it do?

Glutamate, Headaches and Migraines, Oh My!

You know it well. A hard day at work has ended and you are looking forward to that time to unwind. The kids have come home from school, already whining about what's for supper. Your spouse just opened the mail and four more bills are overdue. The dog just threw up on the carpet...again.

The throbbing starts, nagging at first. Getting stronger and stronger until the pounding hammers in your ears. You want to clamp a pillow over your head, but instead manage to lurch into the

---

[62] http://www.ajinomoto.co.jp/ajinomoto/A-Life/e_aminoscience/bc/amino_07.html.

bathroom to grab the strongest headache medication you can find. Tossing back a couple tablets you can hardly wait for the pain to stop.

Headaches are one of the most common illnesses in America. It is rare that a family can go without using pain medication to counteract their frequency. The age of people getting headaches has dropped dramatically. Now even five year olds complain of headaches.

For those with migraines, the symptoms are far worse. Severe migraine affects more than 28 million Americans. A medication that can prevent migraines has not yet been found.[63] The pain can be so bad that the victim becomes sick to their stomach. Often lasting for days, migraines can incapacitate otherwise healthy people. Just why have headaches and migraines become an epidemic in today's world? Is it stress, high blood pressure, pollution?

A 2002 study by Diamond & Wenzel stated that migraines manifest themselves with problems affecting the neurological, gastrointestinal and autonomic functions of the body in combination.[64] Could there be a trigger that affects all of these body systems at the same time? This mystery trigger may be the key to unlocking the cause of migraines.

Could it be............ MSG?

> Neurological: Higher blood flow can increase the permeability of membranes allowing for higher Glutamate levels that could cause Glutamate-induced neurotoxicity.

[63] Wheeler, SD. "Anti-epileptic Drug Therapy in Migraine Headache." **Curr Treat Options Neurol** 2002 Sep;4(5):383-394.

[64] Diamond, S. Wenzel, R. "Practical approaches to migraine management." **Headache** 2003 Mar;43(3):304.

> Gastrointestinal: Ingestion of MSG directly stimulates sites within the gastrointestinal canal.[65]

> Autonomic: Variations in Glutamate within the spinal cord (Central Nervous System) can cause changes in nerve cell membranes, possibly making them more receptive to pain signals.[66]

It appears that MSG could fulfill all three roles that Diamond & Wenzel identified. Glutamate can affect the brain, central nervous system, and digestive system all at the same time.

If MSG does cause headache and migraine, wouldn't there be proof? Plenty!

MSG has been established as a trigger for headaches. Even the FDA admits that headaches are a side effect of eating MSG. A study by the Northern California Headache Clinic showed that chronic headache sufferers decreased the frequency of their headaches simply by reducing their intake of MSG and Hydrolyzed Vegetable Protein (which contains 10-30% MSG).[67]

Sands, Newman, and Lipton of the Albert Einstein College of Medicine in New York also identified Monosodium Glutamate as a leading trigger of headaches. They suggested that avoiding MSG could prevent headaches.[68] In a study of 201 subjects, it was discovered that 28.8% of them had Glutamate-induced headaches. The study went on to say that these headaches could indicate damage to the central nervous system.[69]

---

[65] Niijima, A. "Reflex effects of oral, gastrointestinal and hepatoportal Glutamate sensors on vagal nerve activity." **J Nutr** 2000 Apr;130(4S Suppl):971S-3S.

[66] Devulder, J. Crombez, E. Mortier, E. "Central pain: an overview." **Acta Neurol Belg** 2002 Sep;102(3):97-103.

[67] Scopp AL. "MSG and hydrolyzed vegetable protein induced headache: review and case studies."**Headache**,1991,Feb;31(2):107-10.

[68] Sands, GH. Newman, L. Lipton, R. "Cough, exertional, and other miscellaneous headaches." **Med Clin North Am** 1991 May;75(3):733-47.

[69] Pokras, RS. "A possible role of Glutamate in the aging process." **Med Hypotheses** 1994 Apr;42(4):253-6.

High Glutamate content within the spinal cord can also induce headaches. Both chronic tension headaches[70] and chronic daily headaches can be linked to Glutamate reactions within the Central Spinal Fluid. [71] Both headaches and migraines in children have been linked to Monosodium Glutamate in the diet. Treatment of these disorders should include avoidance of the dietary trigger.[72]

The toxicity of MSG seems to be directly related to how much food you ingest with the additive, and how long you go without eating food afterwards. Researchers have shown that 100% of people who ate MSG laced foods and then fasted overnight complained of headaches.[73]

Hopefully those of you that suffer from headaches and migraines, or have children who do, will benefit from the evidence gathered by these devoted researchers. If your symptoms are triggered by MSG sensitivity, the best way to test for it is to experiment on you and your own family by avoiding all foods that contain MSG or MSG related ingredients.

After the terrible shock that we all suffered in September of 2001, my family sought solace by turning to comfort foods. In the months that followed almost all of our meals were coming out of drive-through windows, or microwave friendly packaging. Not only did our weight increase, so too did the incidence of headaches. Even our children suffered from headaches on frequent basis. We were going through pain relief pills in such numbers that we started buying the jumbo-sized bottles.

---

[70] Sarchielli, P, Alberti, A. Floridi, A. Gallai, V. "L-Arginine/nitric oxide pathway in chronic tension-type headache: relation with serotonin content and secretion and Glutamate content." **J Neurol Sci** 2002 Jun 15;198(1-2):9-15.

[71] Gallai, V. Alberti, A. Gallai, B. Coppola, F. Floridi, A. Sarchielli, P. "Glutamate and nitric oxide pathway in chronic daily headache: evidence from cerebrospinal fluid." **Cephalalgia** 2003 Apr;23(3):166-74.

[72] Millichap, JG. Yee, MM. "The diet factor in pediatric and adolescent migraine." **Pediatr Neurol** 2003 Jan;28(1):9-15.

[73] Chadami, H. Kumar, S. Abaci, F. "Studies on Monosodium Glutamate Ingestion: Biochemical Exploration of Chinese Restaurant Syndrome." **Biochemical Medicine**. 5(1971): 447-456.

All that changed when we discovered the dangers of MSG. Boxed, canned and frozen foods laced with MSG were taken out of our cupboards, fridge, and pantry. Items at fast food restaurants that contained Glutamates were now avoided. Within weeks of altering our diet we noticed a considerable change. The bottle of headache pain reliever was no longer a daily visitor at our table. In fact, it has disappeared to the back of the medicine cabinet, hidden behind the bandages. From February of 2002, to the time of penning this book, our family has been headache free. Head pain that used to be a part of our daily life is now only a memory.

Could it be that easy for your family? It wouldn't hurt to try. The rewards of living pain free are definitely worth the price of giving up MSG laced fried chicken and gravy.

ADHD, Epidemic in Our Schools

The principal sat behind her desk, disgusted. Yet again this boy stood before her, yet again he had disrupted the classroom and been sent down to her office. Yet again he had assaulted another student and required teacher intervention. This time, however, it had taken three teachers to hold him down. Something had to be done.

The written list of complaints the teacher reported to her read like a rap sheet:

- ➢ Short attention span, easily distracted.
- ➢ Constantly moving.
- ➢ Shows no interest when others are talking.
- ➢ Trouble waiting – usually gets in fights at this time.
- ➢ Cannot stay seated.

- ➤ Does not comply with instructions.
- ➤ Has problems with his school work.
- ➤ Easily distracted.
- ➤ Draws on other people's papers.
- ➤ Will not line up – just runs around.
- ➤ Complains of being bored.
- ➤ Spends a lot of time on time-out chair because of not listening or breaking rules or fighting.
- ➤ Does not respond to a reward system, no matter how simple.

This boy was trouble, and she had more just like him. He just wasn't cut out for her school. She called in the parent and handed over the list of complaints. Careful not to call it 'suspension" she told the parent that the boy couldn't be served in her school. Maybe next year he might grow out of it, and could come back.

The parent listened to the professional opinion of the educator, got the boy's things, and together they left the school. Who knew that Kindergarten could be such a tough year?

This boy isn't alone, there are more than a million like him in the schools of United States and Canada, and their numbers are growing every year.

Attention Deficit Hyperactive Disorder (ADHD) is quickly becoming the most prevalent problem with young students today. The National Institute of Mental Health states that about 3% of school children now have ADHD, and that number is growing. The occurrence of ADHD has increased 500 percent in the last decade, and shows no signs of slowing down. At this growth rate, in only twenty years 75% of all school-aged children will have ADHD. Are they doomed to suffer the same fate as the kindergarten student?

ADHD strikes more often in boys (75%) then in girls. It is a disorder that alters the victim globally, affecting their entire personality and demeanor. Children with ADHD grow into adults with ADHD. The problems they have in youth may hamper them throughout their entire lives.

The medical community is baffled. As yet no cause has been found. Pharmaceutical companies, however, have no end of drugs to offer exhausted parents. Ritalin is the drug of choice. Its long list of side effects is countered by the calm it seems to bring to these children.

ADHD is a condition present at birth. For years, professionals have pointed to its prevalence in families to prove it has a hereditary link.

What if the answer was simpler? Perhaps it isn't a family gene, but rather the similar environment within families that is increasing the disorder faster than the affected generation can replicate itself.

Pregnant woman are becoming more and more concerned about what they are putting into their bodies. They watch their fat intake, cholesterol intake, sugar intake, but no one has ever told them to mind their Glutamate intake. Considering the importance that doctors now place on expectant mothers to take just the right amount of vitamins and folic acid, one would think they would consider carefully what large amounts of brain-altering amino acids could do. There are about twenty amino acids that the human body uses to make proteins. These proteins form all of our organs, tissues and especially brain.

Everything an expectant mother eats can also be consumed by the child growing within her. This is especially true in the first trimester of growth, when the placental barrier that regulates the flow of toxins to the fetus is not fully developed. The placental barrier is designed to allow amino acids into the fetus to make the body tissues and organs. Researchers have found that not only do amino acids cross the barrier to the baby, but they also tend to collect there so that the concentration of these chemicals is higher in the growing fetus than in the mother's blood.[74] This can become especially dangerous when the mother eats food containing MSG. Dr. J.W. Olney, a specialist in MSG research at the Department of Psychiatry, Washington University School of Medicine, Missouri, discovered that MSG in the diet of pregnant primates causes brain damage in the offspring.[75] Dr. Olney has since continued to expand on his research of the effects of MSG on subjects and discovered that:

> *"the human food supply is a source of excitotoxins that can damage the brain by one type of mechanism to which immature consumers are hypervulnerable, or by other mechanisms to which adult and elderly consumers are peculiarly sensitive."[76]*

If large amounts of MSG gather within the developing fetus, the increased state of Glutamate excitotoxicity could alter the brain itself in the developing stage. Neuronal pathways growing in the developing brain could be excited into greater, more rapid development.

The brain could become over-simulated so that some areas could become hyper-sensitized to Glutamate, while others could be overdeveloped to the point of cellular death.

ADHD infants show susceptibility to high levels of Glutamate within their neuronal regions.[77] If Glutamate in utero can over-develop neuronal pathways in the fetal brain, perhaps that would explain the hyperactive difficulties in the ADHD child after birth.

---

[74] Kerr, GR. Waisman, HA. "Transplacental ratios of serum-free amino acids during pregnancy in Rhesus monkeys." In Amino Acid Metabolism and Genetic Variation edited by Nathal, WL. New York: McGraw Hill, 1967. pp 429-437.

[75] Olney, JW. "Toxic effects of Glutamate and related amino acids on the developing central nervous system." Inheritable Disorders of Amino Acid Metabolism, edited by Nylan, WN. New York: John Wiley and Sons, 1974, pp 501-511.

[76] Olney, JW. "Excitotoxins in foods." **Neurotoxicology** 1994 Fall;15(3):535-44.

[77] Lou, HC. "Etiology and pathogenesis of attention-deficit hyperactivity disorder (ADHD): significance of prematurity and perinatal hypoxic-haemodynamic encephalopathy." **Acta Paediatr** 1996 Nov;85(11):1266-71.

Researchers at the Department of Psychiatry, Dalhousie University in Halifax, Nova Scotia, used proton magnetic resonance spectroscopy to compare normal children's brain chemistry to that of ADHD children. After measuring a number of chemical reactions in the brains, they discovered that the only difference they found in brain chemistry between ADHD and normal children was the elevated Glutamate levels.[78]

If higher Glutamate levels in ADHD children were reduced in the diet, could the symptoms of the disorder be reduced? Yes. Research shows that parents who place their children on a low MSG diet can reduce the frequency of negative behaviors associated with the disorder.[79] ADHD is a relatively new disorder. It has a very short history and has been noticed and diagnosed only within the last 50 years. In the 1970's it was loosely identified as hyperactivity, in the 80's it was labeled Attention Deficit Hyperactivity Disorder.

ADHD's dramatic increase in cases coincides directly with the introduction of MSG in mass marketed foods in America. The dramatic increase in ADHD cases seems to correlate directly with our increased consumption of restaurant and pre processed foods.

MSG intake could be the very cause of the ADHD that is now rampant in our children. If the current growth pattern of ADHD continues, soon these children will make up the majority in the classroom, and the adult population as well.

---

[78] MacMaster, FP. Carrey, N. Sparkes, S. Kusumakar, V. "Proton spectroscopy in medication-free pediatric attention-deficit/hyperactivity disorder." **Biol Psychiatry** 2003 Jan 15;53(2):184-7.

[79] Kaplan, BJ. McNicol, J. Conte, RA. Moghadam, HK. "Dietary replacement in preschool-aged hyperactive boys." **Pediatrics** 1989 Jan;83(1):7-17.

Autism: the Dumbing of America

ADHD is not the only disorder that is exploding in our nations' youth. Autism is a form of mental disability that is growing in frequency and severity.

Autism is an ailment that manifests as the retardation of the mental abilities of the victim. Children with the disorder can have extreme anti-social behaviors, act abusive to others or themselves, practice continual repetitive motion, show delayed and reduced language development and use, as well as other socially unacceptable behaviors. A few with autism are mildly affected, and can lead almost normal lives. Some have even been noted to have areas of genius. Known as savants, these individuals can have extreme disability in one area, speech for example, while also having incredible ability and innate talent, for instance mathematics or playing an instrument. It seems some areas of their brains can be underdeveloped, while a few have specific areas of exceptional development. Most victims tend to have such severe communication and behavioral problems that society will have to provide them with a lifetime of specialized care.

Autism shares a number of similarities with ADHD. Historically, it was only discovered in the 1940's and then in only a few very rare cases. It is a disorder that develops in the fetus during pregnancy. It is found to occur more often within the same family. Similar to ADHD, individuals with autism are also 75% Male, 25% female. Even more astounding is that the frequency of autism in births has increased 500% in the last decade, just like ADHD.

The research on autism has surprising similarities to that involving ADHD. Many reports on autism refer to discoveries that individuals with the disorder have extreme Glutamate level abnormalities[80] and Glutamate receptor anomalies within the brain.[81]

If MSG intake in the mothers diet during pregnancy is the key to both ADHD and autism, what decides whether a child becomes ADHD or autistic?

It could be possible that the high levels of Glutamate in the developing brain create an over-abundance of Glutamate receptor neurons. With an overabundance of these cells in certain areas of the brain, it could result in the hyperactivity seen in ADHD individuals.

However, if Glutamate levels become too high, excitotoxicity could result, causing the death and destruction of developing neural pathways in the brain. Entire brain regions such as Brocca's area (linked to speech) or other susceptible cells could be stimulated to death, causing that part of the individuals brain to be completely unusable. This kind of global damage could explain the brain abnormalities we see in people with autism. Family genetics may come into play in determining how much MSG it takes to affect the developing fetus.

Reducing MSG in the diet of autistic individuals may not undo the damage done, but it may reduce some of the severity of the autistic symptoms, i.e. self-abuse or repetitive motion.

Hopefully we can reduce the incidence of autism. In 1992, there were 12,000 cases reported in American schools. In 2000 the number ballooned to 80,000.

---

[80] Fatemi, SH. Halt, AR. Stary, JM. Kanodia, R. Schulz, SC. Realmuto, GR. "Glutamic acid decarboxylase 65 and 67 kDa proteins are reduced in autistic parietal and cerebellar cortices." Biol Psychiatry 2002 Oct 15;52(8):805-10.

[81] Jamain, S. Betancur, C. Quach, H. Philippe, A. Fellous, M. Giros, B. Gillberg, C. Leboyer, M. Bourgeron, T. "Linkage and association of the Glutamate receptor 6 gene with autism." Mol Psychiatry 2002;7(3):302-10.

At this rate of increase, by 2008 the population will be a staggering half million cases, and by 2016, 4 million autistic children will require the intensive services of the nation.

By removing MSG and the additives that contain MSG from the diet of pregnant mothers, is it possible that the epidemic of ADHD and autistic children could come to an end?

Something must be done, the sooner, the better.

Schizophrenia

Schizophrenia is a mental disorder whose frequency is also on the rise. People diagnosed with this disorder exhibit signs of brain dysfunction from hallucinations to episodes of mania.

Recent research shows that the common link between people with schizophrenia is an imbalance of brain chemistry, specifically a defect involving the Glutamatergic system.[82] People with this disorder are not able to process Glutamate in the same way that the unafflicted populace does.

It has been suggested that the reduced ability of the brain to transmit Glutamate results in the disturbed information process that is seen in the schizophrenic population.[83]

Studies cited previously in this book have illustrated that excess Glutamate, specifically MSG, can excite neuronal cells to death. Once these cells are killed they cannot be replaced. The ability of MSG to kill Glutamate receptive brain cells could lead to a dramatic reduction in Glutamatergic receptor cells in the brain.

---

[82] Glenthoj, BY. Hemmingsen, R. "Dopaminergic sensitization: implications for the pathogenesis of schizophrenia." **Prog Neuropsychopharmacol Biol Psychiatry** 1997 Jan;21(1):23-46.

[83] Bleich, S. Bleich, K. Wiltfang, J. Maler, JM. Kornhuber, J. "Glutamatergic neurotransmission in schizophrenics." **Fortschr Neurol Psychiatr** 2001 Sep;69 Suppl 2:S56-61.

This reduction could be reflected in the schizophrenic brain's inability to handle Glutamate transmission properly.

Forensic studies of schizophrenic brains show "alterations in Glutamate receptors."[84]

If you were diagnosed with schizophrenia and knew that Glutamate could exacerbate your symptoms, would you approve of its uncontrolled addition to foods?

People with high blood pressure are told to avoid sodium. Why shouldn't schizophrenic people prone to the toxic effects of Glutamate be warned to avoid MSG?

Epilepsy

Michael was a charming man. He was friendly to everyone he met. Always quick with a smile and to offer a hug. He could speak both English and French fluently. No written word was too hard for him to read. Yet when I met him, he was almost forty and still had not learned to drive a car. Michael was mentally handicapped and lived in a group home. He never walked outside unsupervised and had to hold a hand while crossing the street. Michael was autistic, perhaps one of the first people whose autism may have been caused by MSG.

I knew him for five years, and grew to love him with all his habits and idiosyncrasies. As he aged he developed epilepsy. They were small seizures at first, and months would pass between them. But soon they became more serious. His body would shake; he would lose consciousness; and on a few occasions, lost the ability to breathe. Although he had an excellent constitution and rarely even

---

[84] Tsai, G. Coyle, JT. "Glutamatergic mechanisms in schizophrenia." **Annu Rev Pharmacol Toxicol** 2002;42:165-79.

had a cold, the seizures took their toll. Late one night a violent epileptic fit took hold of him. At only 43 he passed away.

People with epilepsy have episodes where they lose mental and bodily control. It can be as inconspicuous as a blank stare (Generalized absence seizure), or as violent as a full body seizure (Tonic-clonic). A misfiring of the brain's nerves causes these seizures. Epilepsy can be a life long condition. It strikes one percent of the population, and affects children and the elderly more often then anyone else. In the majority of cases, the cause of the disability is unknown. Equally mysterious are the factors that trigger the seizures.

Thanks to medical research, epilepsy may not be a mystery forever. Currently, most epilepsy is kept in check by anti-convulsant drugs. Many of these drugs have dangerous side effects when taken long term. Two novel approaches are being taken to reduce seizures in people with epilepsy. One is surgical in nature, referred to as VNS or vagus nerve stimulation, the other is a very restrictive diet known to as the ketogenic diet.

In VNS, an electrical pulse generator is implanted under the skin. It sends out electrical signals to the vagus nerve to reduce the frequency of epileptic seizures. Doctors are not certain why the VNS system is successful, but scientists have found that people helped by this implant have a large reduction in Glutamate within their central nervous systems.[85] MSG is known to over stimulate many organs and tissues within the human body, perhaps the vagus nerve is yet another site where the excitotoxic affects of MSG could induce a harmful response in the body; namely epilepsy.

In the case of the ketogenic diet, people with epilepsy (notably children) are given a strict diet that contains no refined sugar, small servings of fruits and vegetables, and large amounts of fatty foods. Most of the foods on this diet are not the pre-made processed kind,

---

[85] Ben-Menachem, E. Hamberger, A. Hedner, T. Hammond, EJ. Uthman, BM. Slater, J. Treig, T. Stefan, H. Ramsay, RE. Wernicke, JF. et al. "Effects of vagus nerve stimulation on amino acids and other metabolites in the CSF of patients with partial seizures." **Epilepsy Res** 1995 Mar;20(3):221-7.

and are made from scratch in the home. Currently doctors think that it is the low sugar content of the diet that is the reason for the diet's success. In reality, research has not conclusively proven a link between high sugar blood levels and the onset of epileptic seizures.

The ketogenic diet may succeed by reducing MSG in the diet. Because the meal plan does not include factory prepared foods, it is unlikely that the people preparing it are adding the MSG, hydrolyzed plant protein, autolyzed yeast extract or soy protein isolate that can be found in the ready made foods from the grocery store or fast food restaurant. The low levels of Glutamate in the ketogenic diet may be the key to the diet's success, not the decrease in sugar.

While a reduction in sugar may not be the reason the ketogenic diet succeeds, sugar levels do have something to do with epileptic seizures observed in newborns. This has been observed in cases where newborn human infants were hyperinsulinaemic.[86] You may remember this term, it is what MSG treated neonatal rats develop. The insulin levels in their blood are so high that their blood sugar levels drop to dangerous levels. In human infants, this hyperinsulinaemia can result in full body convulsions. Perhaps it is MSG that causes epilepsy in new born children due to an abnormally low blood sugar level.

MSG has also been found to create epileptic seizures in the brain. Scientific researchers turn to their MSG suppliers like Ajinomoto Corporation for their much-needed epilepsy causing excitotoxins. MSG is used with regularity in animal studies when scientists want to induce epileptic seizures.[87] One study found that the severity of epileptic seizures in rats that was produced by commercial MSG

---

[86] Semiz, S. Bircan, I. Akcurin, S. Mihci, E. Melikoglu, M. Karaguzel, G. Kilicaslan, B. Karpuzoglu, G. "Persistent hyperinsulinaemic hypoglycaemia of infancy: case report." **East Afr Med J** 2002 Oct;79(10):554-6.

[87] Feria-Velasco, A. Feria-Cuevas, Y. Gutierrez-Padilla, R. "Chronobiological variations in the convulsive effect of monosodium L-Glutamate when administered to adult rats." Arch Med Res 1995;26 Spec No:S127-32.

increased as the subjects age. The seizures became more tonic-clonic as the animals grow older. The chance of seizure causing death is also increased.[88] Human epilepsy has a similar pattern. Children show more generalized absence seizures, while the elderly show more tonic-clonic types. Elderly humans have the greater chance of epileptic seizure resulting in death.

No matter how one looks at it, the research is plentiful and shocking: *"Monosodium L-Glutamate (MSG), a commonly used food additive, induces convulsive disorders in rats."*[89] Even more alarming is that this discovery was made in 1975, yet nowhere at the FDA did alarm bells go off.

Through all of this, I can't help but think of Michael. Not only could MSG have caused lifelong affliction, it could have been the cause of his death as well.

Alzheimer's Disease

Not everyone that eats MSG becomes obese and diabetic. As we have seen in the chapter on obesity, there may be a predisposition for those ailments caused by large amounts of MSG during the early stages of growth. What about people who are not over-exposed to MSG in youth? Are they safe from its toxic affects?

Perhaps not.

---

[88] Arauz-Contreras, J. Feria-Velasco, A. "Monosodium-L-Glutamate-induced convulsions--I. Differences in seizure pattern and duration of effect as a function of age in rats." **Gen Pharmacol** 1984;15(5):391-5.

[89] Nemeroff, CB. Crisley, FD. "Monosodium L-Glutamate-induced convulsions: temporary alteration in blood-brain barrier permeability to plasma proteins." **Environ Physiol Biochem** 1975;5(6):389-95.

MSG even affects normal people when they eat it. The ingested MSG over-stimulates the pancreas, causing large amounts of insulin to be created.[90] [91] This insulin acts to lower the sugar level in the blood. In diabetics the pancreas becomes so over-stimulated that it fails. In some people, an over-stimulated pancreas can continue creating large amounts of insulin their entire lives. Though these people are spared from diabetes, they are candidates for another terrible disease: Alzheimer's.

Dr. Russell Blaylock, author of *Excitotoxins The Taste that Kills,* makes a compelling argument that Alzheimer's and MSG intake are closely linked. Dr. Blaylock points out that glucose is essential for protecting the brain from excess Glutamate that can excite neuronal cells to death.[92]

When rats are fed MSG and glucose at the same time, they show less brain damage than rats that eat MSG alone.[93] The availability of extra glucose allows the brain to protect itself from the ravages of excitotoxins like MSG.

Dr. Blaylock goes on to establish a link between the low blood sugar levels in aging populations and Alzheimer's disease. He also points out that Alzheimer's patients are more reactive to glucose than the rest of the population, showing lower blood sugar and higher levels of insulin.

In a 1983 study by Bucht, Adolfsson, Lithner, and Winblad, 839 psychiatric patients were examined. Of the 839, 63 were diabetic. Of these diabetic patients, not one had dementia due to

---

[90] Graham, TE. Sgro, V. Friars, D. Gibala, MJ. "Glutamate ingestion: the plasma and muscle free amino acid pools of resting humans." **Am J Physiol Endocrinol Metab** 2000 Jan;278(1):E83-9

[91] Mourtzakis, M. Graham, TE. "Glutamate ingestion and its effects at rest and during exercise in humans." **J Appl Physiol** 2002 Oct;93(4):1251-9.

[92] Blaylock, Dr. Russell. Excitotoxins: The Taste that Kills. Health Press, 1997. Pg 159.

[93] Henneberry, R.C. "The role of Neuronal energy in the neurotoxicity of excitatory amino acids." **Neurobiology of Aging** 10(1989):611-613.

Alzheimer's, leading the researchers to the conclusion that diabetes may not co-exist with Alzheimer's disease.[94]

Do diabetics get Alzheimer's disease?

Two independent studies, one done at Albert Einstein College of Medicine in New York, the other done at University of California's Institute for Brain Aging and Dementia, looked at populations of elderly patients. Both studies came to the conclusion that patients with diabetes are not at risk for Alzheimer's disease and that the two conditions existing together are extremely rare.[95] [96] Here we are, with two of the most prevalent and destructive diseases that affect the elderly. This book has already illustrated how MSG can cause diabetes, would you be surprised if it caused Alzheimer's as well?

The research is convincing.

The symptoms of Alzheimer's are caused by neural damage in the hippocampus and basal forebrain. These structures have a great deal to do with memory. Research done at the Laboratory of Neurosciences, National Institute on Aging, Baltimore, Maryland, supports the idea that the key feature that may cause Alzheimer's is the imbalance between glucose and Glutamate in the brain. Five other studies done at the University of Kentucky, U.S.A., University Medical School, Switzerland, and the Heidelburg University in Germany have all come to similar findings.[97 98 99 100 101]

---

[94] Bucht, G. Adolfsson, R. Lithner, F. Winblad, B. "Changes in blood glucose and insulin secretion in patients with senile dementia of Alzheimer type." **Acta Med Scand** 1983;213(5):387-92.

[95] Heitner, J. Dickson, D. "Diabetics do not have increased Alzheimer-type pathology compared with age-matched control subjects. A retrospective postmortem immunocytochemical and histofluorescent study." **Neurology 1997** Nov;49(5):1306-11.

[96] Nielson, KA. Nolan, JH. Berchtold, NC. Sandman, CA. Mulnard, RA. Cotman, CW. "Apolipoprotein-E genotyping of diabetic dementia patients: is diabetes rare in Alzheimer's disease?" **J Am Geriatr Soc** 1996 Aug;44(8):897-904.

[97] Smith-Swintosky, VL. Mattson, MP. "Glutamate, beta-amyloid precursor proteins, and calcium mediated neurofibrillary degeneration." **J Neural Transm Suppl** 1994;44:29-45.

[98] Meier-Ruge, W. Bertoni-Freddari, C. "The significance of glucose turnover in the brain in the pathogenetic mechanisms of Alzheimer's disease." **Rev Neurosci** 1996 Jan-Mar;7(1):1-19.

High levels of Glutamate and low levels of glucose cause brain cell destruction in people with Alzheimer's disease (AD). Glucose acts like a police force in the brain, rounding up dangerous groups of harmful substances and arresting their development into deadly gangs. If glucose is not freely available for the brain to maintain safe levels of Glutamate, the increased Glutamate can overwhelm brain neurons and cause cell destruction.

M.P. Mattson et al. at the National Institute on Aging, Baltimore, take it a step further, arguing there is:

> *"Emerging evidence that dietary restriction can forestall the development of AD ...... is consistent with a major "metabolic" component to these disorders, and provides optimism that these devastating brain disorders of aging may be largely preventable."*[102]

The 'metabolic' condition that these scientists speak of bears a striking resemblance to MSG. MSG not only excites the pancreas to keep blood sugar low and less available to the brain, it also makes extra Glutamate available to enter the brain and cause massive cell destruction.

Unfortunately, it seems that people whose pancreases manage to survive the stimulation by MSG that has kept their blood levels in a constant state of sugar starvation face a different problem than

---

[99] Hoyer S. "Oxidative metabolism deficiencies in brains of patients with Alzheimer's disease." **Acta Neurol Scand Suppl** 1996;165:18-24.

[100] Meier-Ruge, WA. Bertoni-Freddari, C. "Pathogenesis of decreased glucose turnover and oxidative phosphorylation in ischemic and trauma-induced dementia of the Alzheimer type." **Ann N Y Acad Sci** 1997 Sep 26;826:229-41.

[101] Mattson, MP. Guo, ZH. Geiger, JD. "Secreted form of amyloid precursor protein enhances basal glucose and Glutamate transport and protects against oxidative impairment of glucose and Glutamate transport in synaptosomes by a cyclic GMP-mediated mechanism." **J Neurochem** 1999 Aug;73(2):532-7.

[102] Mattson, MP. Pedersen, WA. Duan, W. Culmsee, C. Camandola, S. "Cellular and molecular mechanisms underlying perturbed energy metabolism and neuronal degeneration in Alzheimer's and Parkinson's diseases." **Ann N Y Acad Sci** 1999;893:154-75.

diabetes as they age: Alzheimer's. Constant intake of MSG (such as in heavily 'seasoned' institutional food) results in stimulation of the insulin making beta cells. Elevated insulin levels cause the amount of sugar available to the brain to drop, creating a chronic low blood sugar level. Then, as Dr. Blaylock explained, the brain which uses 25% of the body's glucose intake becomes dangerously deprived of glucose. Without glucose to change Glutamate into less toxic substances, the Glutamate is then free to collect in dangerous levels around the brains neurons.[103] Glutamate in high levels causes neuronal cell death.[104] The resulting cell death can manifest itself as Alzheimer's disease.

Why is it that those with diabetes do not get Alzheimer's? People with diabetes have difficulty keeping their blood sugar from being chronically high. They tend to have blood with very high glucose levels, resulting in plenty of sugar for the brain to use to metabolize and equalize Glutamate levels in the brain. It seems the elderly are stricken by two main diseases, Diabetes or Alzheimer's. Monosodium Glutamate may cause both.

Parkinson's and Huntington's Disease

Genes are the blueprint for our bodies. They not only tell our cells just how to replicate, they also allow for differences in people. For some, genes can hold a code that makes them react differently to chemicals than other people. The way they react to these chemicals may determine their level of health.

For some people, Glutamate is such a chemical.

---

[103] Blaylock, Dr. Russell. Excitotoxins: The Taste that Kills. Health Press, 1997. Pg 159.

[104] Bezvenyuk Z, Miettinen R, Solovyan V. "Chromatin condensation during Glutamate-induced excitotoxicity of cerebellar [correction of celebellar] granule neurons precedes disintegration of nuclear DNA into high molecular weight DNA fragments." **Brain Res Mol** 2003 Jan 31;110(1):140-6.

Parkinson's disease manifests itself as the destruction of neurons in the substantia nigra-striatum of the brain. Symptoms of this ailment included rigidity of limbs, tremors, mental dementia, and reduced movement. Recent research on the origins of Parkinson's has found that close relatives of those afflicted have a higher chance of getting it, yet no genetic link has been found. This could support the idea that diet, which families tend to share in similarity, could be a possible cause.

Surprisingly, the brain damage seen in Parkinson's patients mimics the same stress due to failure of the brain to regulate glucose and Glutamate levels that Alzheimer's victims suffer from. The difference in the disorders seems to be in the area of the brain that suffers from cellular death.[105]

If the key to Alzheimer's is the low glucose availability in brain's blood sugar caused by ingestion of MSG, there could also be a link between MSG and Parkinson's disease.

The connection of brain diseases with MSG does not end here.

Huntington's disease is a genetic disorder that affects people as they age. The brain degenerates and causes the victim such problems as reduction in cognitive ability, poor body control, forgetfulness, depression, twitching of limbs, and other symptoms, which can lead to an untimely death.

A 2002 study at the University of Freiburg, Germany, it was discovered that the mutant Huntington gene causes a:

> *"progressively deranged Glutamate handling in the brain, beginning before the onset of symptoms ....provide evidence for a contribution of excitotoxicity to the pathophysiology of Huntington's*

---

[105] Mattson, MP. Pedersen, WA. Duan, W. Culmsee, C. Camandola, S. "Cellular and molecular mechanisms underlying perturbed energy metabolism and neuronal degeneration in Alzheimer's and Parkinson's diseases." **Ann N Y Acad Sci** 1999;893:154-75.

disease, and thus Huntington's disease may be added to the growing list of neurodegenerative disorders associated with compromised Glutamate transport capacity."[106]

The gene in Huntington's disease seems to affect the way the brain processes Glutamate. In Celiac disease, the human body is unable to handle the gluten found in common foods such as wheat products. To these people, even bread can be toxic. Perhaps the same could be said about Huntington's disease and MSG?

If both Parkinson's disease and Huntington's disease are related to high levels of Glutamate in the brain, could eating more and more Glutamate exacerbate these conditions?

Though this hypothesis has yet to be fully explored, there is certainly enough published research to justify further study in this direction.

---

[106] Behrens, PF. Franz, P. Woodman, B. Lindenberg, KS. Landwehrmeyer, GB. "Impaired Glutamate transport and Glutamate-glutamine cycling: downstream effects of the Huntington mutation." **Brain** 2002 Aug;125(Pt 8):1908-22.

MSG: Not Just in Chinese Food Anymore

If we just stop eating MSG, maybe we can put a stop to the growing epidemic of obesity, diabetes, ADHD, autism, schizophrenia, epilepsy, Alzheimer's, Huntington's and Parkinson's diseases in today's population.

It's not that easy. MSG is everywhere!

In the last thirty years, the greatest change to the North American diet has come in the form of fast food. Families are eating out twenty times more than they did three decades ago. It is at these fast food establishments that our bodies face undisclosed amounts of MSG.

The food industry wants you to believe that MSG in restaurants is confined to Chinese dining establishments. As recently as 1999, R. Walker, researcher for the Food and Agriculture Organization of the United Nations, referred to Monosodium Glutamate as an ingredient in "ethnic cuisines."[107] We would hardly consider McDonald's to be ethnic cuisine, nor do we think that A&W, Applebee's, Arby's, Big Boy, Bob Evans, Bonanza, Boston Market, Boston Pizza, Burger King, Captain D's, Carls Jr., Chili's, Church's Chicken, Cracker Barrel, Dairy Queen, Denny's, Domino's, Golden Corral, Hard Rock Café, Hardee's, Harvey's,

---

[107] Walker R. "The significance of excursions above the ADI. Case study: Monosodium Glutamate." **Regul Toxicol Pharmacol** 1999 Oct;30(2 Pt 2):S119-21.

Hooters, International House of Pancakes, Jack in the Box, Kentucky Fried Chicken, Long John Silver's, Outback Steakhouse, Pizza Hut, Ponderosa, Popeye's, Red Lobster, Ruby Tuesday, Sizzler, Sonic Drive-In, Swiss Chalet, Taco Bell, T.G.I Friday's, Tim Horton's, Pizzeria Uno, Village Inn, Wendy's, Western Sizzlin, White Castle, or the myriad of other fast food establishments that use large amounts of MSG, hydrolyzed protein or other glutamates in their foods, to be 'ethnic' in their menu offerings.

MSG, once thought of as a seasoning found only in chinese buffets, is now found in almost every restaurant across the continent. Everyday we order from those smiling faces behind the counters. We offer our children a tray filled with items whose origin is unknown, filled with more Glutamate than their bodies need.

In fact, our bodies do not need any MSG, not a bit, not even a gram.

MSG is not a vitamin, mineral, or even a source of nutrition. While Glutamates can be found in nature in small amounts, MSG can be found distilling in giant vats, where bacteria breaks down proteins and excretes Monosodium Glutamate. Here is the industrial origin of MSG in your food (known in manufacturing and laboratories as L-Glutamate). This is what we are putting in our children's bodies:

"Since the discovery of Corynebacterium glutamicum as an efficient Glutamate-overproducing microorganism in 1957, the production of L-amino acids by the fermentative method has become one of the most important research-target of industrial microbiology. Several research groups have developed metabolic engineering principles for L-amino acid-producing C. glutamicum strains over the last four decades. The mechanism of L-Glutamate-overproduction by the microorganism is very unique and interesting. L-Glutamate overproduction by this bacterium, a biotin auxotroph, is induced by a biotin limitation and suppressed by an excess of biotin. Addition of a surfactant or penicillin is known to induce L-Glutamate overproduction under excess biotin. After the development of the general molecular biology tools such as cloning vectors and DNA transfer technique, genes encoding biosynthetic enzymes were isolated.

With those genes and tools, recombinant DNA technology can be applied in analysis of biosynthetic pathways and strain construction of C. glutamicum.[108]

Did the above paragraph make sense to you? It certainly baffles me. This description does not sound like a natural way to make something that we eat on a daily basis. Yet it is the above process that creates the MSG that food manufactures can refer to as "natural flavorings' on food ingredients lists. The Glutamate manufacturers have even managed to get organic associations to consider MSG to be a natural and organic ingredient.

MSG is put in food for two reasons: to make us choose the product that has it over one that doesn't, and to make us eat more of that product.

In 1909, Dr. Ikeda patented the production of this 'natural ingredient,' a flavor he called Unami. Today 1.5 million tons of MSG is produced for the global food industry. 3 billion pounds of flavoring per year are being added to our food. Ajinomoto Company is proud to supply a third of the world's MSG, and claims that the use of MSG grows by 6% every year. Not only does Ajinomoto sell MSG to the food industry, but also to laboratories for use in animal experiments, some of which may have been quoted in this book.

Not the most wholesome thing we would want to give our children, is it?

Maybe you can still go to restaurants; you'll just be sure to ask if there is any MSG in the menu item you would like. Be prepared to practice patience. Some restaurants have a brochure with MSG and other Glutamate containing ingredients like hydrolyzed protein or autolyzed yeast to show you. We appreciate restaurants like this; sadly they are few and far between. We have had more than one restaurant manager swear up and down they didn't use MSG, only to have him or her come out to our table minutes later red

---

[108] **Kimura, E.** Fermentation & Biotechnology Laboratories, Ajinomoto Co., Inc., "Metabolic engineering of Glutamate production." **Adv Biochem Eng Biotechnol** 2003;79:37-57.

faced with an apology. Some establishments have web sites with nutritional information, but they often leave out things like sodium casienate, yeast extract, seasonings, or natural flavorings. Glutamates can be hidden within all of these ingredients. Try to research or call ahead. We have left more restaurants without ordering more times than I care to remember.

Maybe you think you can avoid MSG by staying at home and avoiding the fast food restaurant scene. Just pick up some supplies at the grocery store and make tasty meals at home.

It's not that easy.

MSG in one form or another has found its way into almost every processed food you can think of. MSG isn't always listed on ingredients labels. It could be hidden under the following names and ingredients:

Always Contains MSG:

Monosodium Glutamate
Monopotassium Glutamate   Yeast Extract
Hydrolyzed Protein (any)   Glutamic Acid
Calcium Caseinate   Sodium Caseinate
Yeast Food   Hydrolyzed Corn Gluten
Gelatin   Textured Protein
Yeast Nutrient   Autolyzed Yeast

May contain glutamate, or create it during processing:

Carrageenan   Natural Pork Flavoring
Citric Acid   Maltodextrin
Bouillon and Broth   Natural Chicken Flavor
Natural Beef flavor   Whey Protein Concentrate
Stock   Whey Protein
Ultra Pasteurized   Soy Sauce
Barley Malt   anything Enzyme
Pectin   anything Enzyme Modified

Protease	Malt flavoring
Protease Enzymes	Soy Protein
Soy Protein Isolate	Soy protein concentrate
Whey protein isolate	Malt Extract
anything Fermented	anything Protein Fortified.

and even hidden in Natural Flavors & Seasonings

from 'www.Truthinlabeling.org'

Pick out almost any processed food in a grocery store and it is likely that these glutamate containing ingredients, separately or in combination, are in the mix.

Government agencies like the FDA make it easy for manufacturers to hide MSG under labels like 'seasonings', or 'natural flavorings'. How are parents supposed to buy wholesome products for their children if they aren't properly told what's in them. Be extra careful of products that say 'No added MSG', this statement implies that there is already some in it. Be wary of a seasoning called "Accent" it is 100% MSG in its powder form.

As you can see from this extensive list, there is a lot to remember. Even in our MSG free home, we have purchased products, even "Organically Certified" ones, and found on closer inspection that they have one of these sources of glutamate in them.

Glutamate producers are constantly trying to find new ways to add MSG into people's diets. They have already started promoting the use of MSG as a spray to use on crops (even organic ones) as they grow in the field.

The Truth in Labeling organization has been lobbying the federal government for years trying to get them to close the loop holes to listing MSG as Seasoning and Natural flavoring.

If you are serious about protecting your family from MSG, it will mean a lot of sacrifice. Almost all snack foods, prepared frozen entrees, and prepared meats have one, two, or more of these ingredients. Soups are filled with them, and are especially dangerous as MSG in liquid form raises the Glutamate levels in the blood higher then when taken in powder form. We had hoped to list in this book every brand name grocery item that contained glutamate in some form or another, but after days researching at the grocery stores, the list had grown to two hundred items, and we had only made it down two aisles. Just as the actual legal system starts with the belief that everyone is guilty until proven innocent, when shopping you must apply the same reasoning to every prepared, boxed, and manufactured food item you pick up. If the ingredients list does not have a single item from the list printed in this book, you have no guarantee that you are getting a product without glutamates in it.

Though manufacturers are allowed to put as much MSG in their product as they want, (60% MSG content or more is permissible), it only takes a small amount to affect your brain.

A study in France suggested that at the level of 0.6 %, MSG in food caused people to eat more of it, and faster.[109]   When you consider that the average person in America may eat more than two kg's (app 4 pounds) of MSG laced food a day, that's 12 grams, almost two teaspoons of pure MSG. If MSG makes you eat more, wouldn't it benefit restaurants to add even more than that, perhaps 1-2%? After all, there are no limits under FDA rulings. This is very disconcerting considering it only takes one to two tablespoons to kill a dog. VETSIN (MSG) is used in the Phillipines to kill dogs. The MSG is put in a bread roll and given to the dog, resulting in unconsciousness, convulsions, and then death.[110]

It's time to start reading labels.

As I have stated before, almost every processed food contains added Glutamate in some form or another. Most Glutamate that occurs naturally in foods like tomatoes or mushrooms is bound to

[109] Bellisle, F. Monneuse, MO. Chabert, M. Larue-Achagiotis, C. Lanteaume, MT. Louis-Sylvestre, J. "Monosodium Glutamate as a palatability enhancer in the European diet." **Physiol Behav** 1991 May;49(5):869-73.

[110] Schwartz, Dr. George. In Bad Taste, Health Press, 1999. pg 61.

other amino acids and does not affect the body. Unbound Glutamate found in artificial food additives is another story. MSG is the most common unbound form of glutamate. Some scientists refer to it as a free radical: a highly reactive molecule that wants to attach to something else. With every entrée we eat, we could be overwhelming our pancreases and bringing ourselves one-step closer to a diabetic break down. Children aren't even safe when having school lunches. The latest money saving idea in America's schools is to enter into contracts with fast food establishments to supply the kids with fast food full of MSG in their cafeterias.

Institutions such as retirement homes are seeing an increase in diabetes and Alzheimer's in the elderly. Hospitals and other large facilities often use MSG to make the mass produced meals more palatable. One study done in 1999 actually went as far as to suggest that facilities add MSG to the foods that they feed their elderly and diabetic patients. The study suggested that by adding MSG, dieticians could purposely alter resident's choices of what foods they will eat.[111] MSG sounds more like a drug than a food additive.

We teach our kids, "Say no to drugs", so why are we feeding this to them?

---

[111] Bellisle, F. "Effects of Monosodium Glutamate on human food palatability." **Ann N Y Acad Sci** 1998 Nov 30;855:438-41.

MSG Safety: The Great Deception

A drug is any chemical used to create a desired physiological affect in the body. In medical laboratories, we have seen how MSG is used to make mice populations obese and to kill specific areas of the brain. The scientists who produce these studies value MSG as a drug, not as a harmless food additive.

MSG is a drug, one of the most potent drugs in your body. It affects your body in the same manner that pharmaceuticals do.

The companies that create MSG know that it has a great deal of value in medical research. Ajinomoto Company, the world's largest producer and supplier of MSG, sells L-Glutamate (MSG) to the scientific world for use in medical research. Other companies that produce MSG, as well as the food manufacturers that use it, are also well aware of the myriad of affects that MSG has on your body.

In 1909, Dr. Ikeda, inventor of MSG, and patent holder of the process to make it, helped start the Ajinomoto Company. This company prides itself in expanding the use of MSG in products throughout the world.

One of the reasons that the FDA says that MSG is safe is the accepted idea that Glutamate cannot cross the blood brain barrier. If it would only visit the Ajinomoto web site that sells MSG (glutamic acid), and glutamine (Glutamate bonded to ammonia), they would see the companies claim that Glutamine CAN cross the blood brain barrier, and that it can be broken down into Glutamate and ammonia molecules. The Ajinomoto Company itself declares just how Glutamate can enter the brain from the blood stream. Once in the brain, the high levels of Glutamate cause "neuronal suicide."[112]

Interestingly enough the Ajinomoto Website www.ajinomoto.com declares that they have discovered a drug that can be used to counteract diabetes. Not surprising considering they create the MSG that may be the leading cause of diabetes.

How convenient would it be if a company sold both the cause of a disease and its cure?

The Glutamate Association is a government lobby group formed in 1977. Its members include MSG manufactures, as well as food producers that use MSG. The Glutamate Association was created to promote the use of MSG and 'debunk' any research that puts MSG in a negative light.

The Glutamate Association tries to make itself out to be an impartial group that is dispelling the bad publicity and reputation that MSG has received over the years. Impartial, sure. Imagine a nicotine association with tobacco companies as members. Would you believe them if they said, "smoking is actually good for you."

On the Glutamate Association web page, with the misleading name of 'www.msgfacts.com', the 'facts' are presented to support the large-scale use of MSG in the nations food supply.

---

[112] Olney, JW. "New insights and new issues in developmental neurotoxicology." **Neurotoxicology** 2002 Dec;23(6):659-68.

To the question: Does MSG affect metabolism? The Glutamate Association's answer is "No." They have ignored the data at the U.S. National Library of Medicine, where countless journals state in hundreds of experiments that MSG creates obesity. They have overlooked the data from studies showing that even in average people, MSG intake can triple the levels of insulin in the human body.[113]

Perhaps they believe that increased insulin, which creates fat deposits in the body, has nothing to do with metabolism.

The Glutamate Association and its members rebuke and ignore any study that could possibly tarnish their presentation of MSG as the most friendly and benign of food additives, comparing it to baking soda and vinegar. Last I checked vinegar wasn't a key chemical utilized in the brain or the pancreas, and baking soda wasn't used to poison dogs.

When the association explains the reason that MSG should be added to food, they offer the excuse that it makes food taste good, and that it is a beneficial way to get the elderly who have depleted taste sensation to eat more food. The Glutamate Association also says that MSG helps people eat less salt. If it makes people eat larger helpings, they would in fact be eating more salt in the extra food that MSG drove them to eat.

America's children are not the elderly. They do not need to eat more food, if anything they are eating too much food. America's children are at great risk of becoming obese. MSG is doing its part to help this.

The only benefits that the official association that supports Glutamate can come up with are: 'It makes people eat more food, and less salt.' Are these reasons worth the increased risk of obesity, diabetes, autism, ADHD, Alzheimer's, and other debilitating disease?

---

[113] Graham, TE. Sgro, V. Friars, D. Gibala, MJ. "Glutamate ingestion: the plasma and muscle free amino acid pools of resting humans. **Am J Physiol Endocrinol Metab** 2000 Jan;278(1):E83-9.

MSG is nicotine for food. The Glutamate Association even supports this idea by saying it gets people to eat more. Nicotine gets people to smoke more. Is it any surprise that some people explain their need to overeat as an addiction?

Recent Supreme Court rulings have found tobacco companies at fault for denying that nicotine gave people the urge to keep smoking. MSG gives people the urge to keep eating. Tobacco causes cancer; MSG may cause an even longer list of diseases. What is the difference between the misleading tobacco companies and the MSG producers?

Not only do the manufactures know that it is a harmful drug that affects major body organs, but the Government knows it as well.

In March 2000, a study from the Federal Bureau of Chemical Safety; Health Protection Branch of the Department of Health Canada had this to say about Monosodium Glutamate and the human body:

Glutamate receptors (GluRs) are ubiquitously present in the central nervous system (CNS) as the major mediators of excitatory neurotransmission and excitotoxicity. Neural injury associated with trauma, stroke, epilepsy, and many neurodegenerative diseases such as Alzheimer's, Huntington's, and Parkinson's diseases and amyotrophic lateral sclerosis may be mediated by excessive activation of Glutamate receptors. Neurotoxicity associated with excitatory amino acids encountered in food, such as domoic acid and Monosodium Glutamate, has also been linked to Glutamate receptors......... also present in kidney, liver, lung, spleen, and testis. Further investigations are needed to assess the role of these receptors in peripheral tissues and their importance in the toxicity of excitatory compounds. Therefore, food safety assessment and neurobiotechnology focusing on drugs designed to interact with Glutamate receptors should consider these tissues as potential target/effector sites.[114]

The Canadian government's Bureau of Chemical Safety recognizes the danger of Monosodium Glutamate. The Bureau refers to MSG as a neurotoxic excitatory amino acid that can stimulate a variety of organs in the body and could be linked to many serious diseases. The Bureau suggests that manufacturers of any drugs that could interact with Glutamate receptors should consider the effects on other tissues, while it ignores the MSG already in our food supply affecting the bodily tissues of the nation.

What has the Canadian government done about the MSG that they have identified as neurotoxic to the human body?

Nothing.

The Canadian Food Inspection Agency (CFIA) has not even put MSG on their allergy alert list. They must have ignored the FDA's report that MSG is a known allergen for an unknown percentage of the population. Instead of listing MSG as a possibly reactive substance (despite the research of their own government.), they instead concentrate on the more dangerous ingredients like soy, sesame seeds and wheat.

The CFIS, just like the American FDA, has done nothing to warn people of the dangers of MSG. The Glutamate Association must be doing an incredible job as a lobby group. It is the prime directive of a lobby group to influence the government in power to make decisions that benefit those the lobby group represent. To date, neither the American, nor the Canadian government have taken heed of the hundreds of reproducible studies that show MSG has detrimental effects to growth and brain activity.

---

[114] Gill, SS. Mueller, RW. McGuire, PF. Pulido, OM. "Potential target sites in peripheral tissues for excitatory neurotransmission and excitotoxicity." **Toxicol Pathol** 2000 Mar-Apr;28(2):277-84. Bureau Chemical Safety, Health Protection Branch, Health Canada, Ottawa, Ontario.

Why would governments defend the Glutamate industry, and protect an additive that could be poisoning their nations. It could well be a case of inherited trouble. MSG was approved by governing bodies that have long since disappeared into antiquity. Does the current one wish to bring light to a blunder even bigger than the fluoride problem they are already covering up? Imagine the lack of credibility the FDA would have if it suddenly did a 180 degree turn to say that the additive it approved and supported in unregulated doses was found to create diabetes, obesity, Alzheimer's, ADHD, autism and other debilitating diseases.

Imagine the backlash against the fast food industry that has been promoting MSG laden bonus size helpings on every man, woman and child in America.

Imagine the repercussions against the food packaging industry that has been using MSG in their products to ensure we would buy more and eat more of their product.

Imagine the loss in revenue of pharmaceutical companies if the key to the cures for diabetes, Alzheimer's and other diseases had more to do with healthy eating than taking a prescribed drug.

In United States, the health industry makes the most money when people are ill. Teaching people to avoid toxins that could make them sick would undercut the profits of the industry.

For all our technology and knowledge, a higher percentage of today's population have some form of illness than almost any other time in the recorded history of mankind.

The origins of this increase in illness can be linked to the 2 major factors that have changed the most in the last century: diet and lifestyle.

Some historians trace the fall of the Roman Empire to the use of lead pipes to carry their drinking water. They did not know that something they ingested was toxic to them. So what is our excuse?

The research is in, and the results are undeniable. MSG can cause terrible effects in the body's natural order. A thousand years from now will the children in a classroom half way round the world study the fall of the American empire, and say, "Why did those people poison themselves? They could put a man on the moon but they couldn't protect themselves from their own blinding greed and ignorance?"

What will the answer be? Will we trust the findings of factual research, or the propaganda of associations funded by the makers of the toxins that could prove society's downfall.

Our children deserve better than that. Our children deserve parents who question the safety of everything that goes into their bodies. Our children deserve to eat food without additives designed to give them an unnatural urge to eat more. Our children deserve to grow into adulthood without threat from diabetes, obesity, autism, Alzheimer's, and other debilitating tragedies.

There are two sides to this battle. Those that demand that MSG and ingredients containing it be removed from the nation's food supply, and those who will stand with the profit driven companies that created it, saying that it has value in our foods.

Is the value of MSG in food worth the risk to our health? The deep pockets of the Glutamate industry certainly think so.

Aspartame: MSG's Evil Twin?

Sadly, fluoride and MSG aren't the only skeletons in the governmental closet. Another amino acid has been launched on unsuspecting consumers. Like MSG and fluoride, the damage it can do is extensive, but this additive's origins are even more suspicious.

In 1965, at a research laboratory at G.D. Searles, James Schlatter accidentally discovered Aspartame (Nutrasweet) while working to find a cure for stomach ulcers. By 1975, G.D. Searle had managed to talk the FDA to allow its use as an artificial sweetener, but not a food additive. By 1975, things were going a little sour. It seems that the research G.D. Searle did to prove the safety of Aspartame left out scientific studies that proved it caused tumors and epileptic seizures in monkeys.[115]

In 1975, FDA Commissioner, Dr. Alexander Schmidt appointed a special Task Force to examine G.D. Searle and its testing methods regarding Aspartame. In 1977, the task force found G.D. Searle Company to be fraudulent in their research on the safety of Aspartame. FDA Chief Counsel, Richard Merrill suggested to U.S.

---

[115] Cloninger, MR. Baldwin, RE. "Aspartylphenylalanine methyl ester: a low-calorie sweetener." **Science** 1970 Oct 2;170(953):81-2.

Attorney Sam Skinner that a grand jury be set up to investigate G.D. Searle. Strangely enough, both Skinner, and his later replacement, never brought G.D. Searle to trial. Instead, both of them were hired away from their government positions by G.D. Searle's law firm.

Dr. John Olney the same scientist who researched the dangers of MSG, along with the FDA, managed to bring together a Public Board of Inquiry to investigate the toxicity of Aspartame. In 1980, the board unanimously voted to reject the use of Aspartame until further testing could be done in regards to research indicating that it caused brain tumors.

For a moment, it looked like the world would be protected from Aspartame. G.D. Searle Corporation, however, had an ace up their sleeve. His name was Donald and they had hired him in 1977 as Chief Executive Officer in an attempt to save the economic ruin that threatened to befall them. Donald had extensive government contacts from his time working as a presidential staffer for both Nixon and Ford.

Donald had business savvy, and was well connected. He saw Aspartame for the cash cow that it could be. In 1980, Aspartame's bid for acceptance as a food additive was stifled, but Donald did not give up.

In January of 1981, just after Ronald Reagan brought the Republicans back to the White House, Donald and G. D. Searle put in a new application to the FDA to declare Aspartame safe as a food additive. In March, FDA Commissioner Jere Goyan established a 5-member panel of scientists to review the issues outlined by the 1980 Public Board of Inquiry. A full review would never come to pass. In April, Reagan replaced FDA Commissioner Jere Goyan with Arthur Hull Hayes, Jr. In July, Hayes ignored all previous findings and declared that Aspartame could be added to food. One year later, it became legal to add it to soft drinks.

Aspartame, aka Nutrasweet, made its mark on the world and guaranteed the financial success of Donald's company. Donald must have impressed Reagan, for in 1983 the President named him special envoy to the Middle East. Donald returned from this post in time to oversee the sale of G. D. Searle to Monsonto Company in 1985.

Diet soda was the new drink of popularity. It was used extensively to supply the troops in action during the Gulf War.

If Aspartame's shrouded and questionable history is not enough to raise your eyebrows, maybe you should consider the toxic effects that research has shown that it has on the body.

Lately, research has found problems with Nutrasweet. Even the official Nutrasweet Website, 'www.nutrasweet.com', states that Nutrasweet breaks down in the body to produce methanol. Methanol in turn creates formaldehyde.[116] The formaldehyde created by Aspartame collects in the tissues of the body organs, especially the liver. Scientific research has found that "Aspartame consumption may constitute a hazard."[117]

The American Academy of Clinical Toxicology states that methanol-derived formaldehyde in the body has been linked to nausea, abdominal pain, blindness, and impairment of the central nervous system.[118] Furthermore formaldehyde in drinking water has been proven to create cancerous tumors.[119]

[116] Barceloux, DG. Bond, GR. Krenzelok, EP. Cooper, H. Vale, JA. "American Academy of Clinical Toxicology practice guidelines on the treatment of methanol poisoning." American Academy of Clinical Toxicology Ad Hoc Committee on the Treatment Guidelines for Methanol Poisoning. J Toxicol Clin Toxicol 2002;40(4):415-46.

[117] Trocho, C. Pardo, R. Rafecas, I. Virgili, J. Remesar, X. Fernandez-Lopez, JA. "Alemany M.Formaldehyde derived from dietary Aspartame binds to tissue components in vivo." Life Sci 1998;63(5):337-49.

[118] Barceloux, DG. Bond, GR. Krenzelok, EP. Cooper, H. Vale, JA. "American Academy of Clinical Toxicology practice guidelines on the treatment of methanol poisoning." American Academy of Clinical Toxicology Ad Hoc Committee on the Treatment Guidelines for Methanol Poisoning. J Toxicol Clin Toxicol 2002;40(4):415-46.

[119] Soffritti, M. Belpoggi, F. Lambertin, L. Lauriola, M. Padovani, M. Maltoni, C. "Results of long-term experimental studies on the carcinogenicity of formaldehyde and acetaldehyde in rats." Ann N Y Acad Sci 2002 Dec;982:87-105.

Formaldehyde is a dangerous chemical that has been shown to cause reactions in many people. Chemical Sensitivity Disorder can be caused by formaldehyde. This disorder may be closely linked to Chronic Fatigue Syndrome, and fibromyalgia.[120]

Chronic Fatigue Syndrome is an ailment on the increase in the nation. Its cause is a mystery to the medical community. One of the main symptoms of CFS is fibromyalgia: chronic pain and soreness in the muscles. Research has shown that human subjects diagnosed with fibromyalgia managed to completely or almost completely reduce the symptoms of the disorder by removing MSG and Aspartame from their diet.[121] If removing these two excitotoxins from the diet can cure fibromyalgia, could they be the cause?

Some people have suggested that in hot conditions (above 86 degrees Fahrenheit) Nutrasweet breaks down to create even higher concentrations of methanol and formaldehyde. Imagine what could happen if diet sodas containing Aspartame were left out in very hot temperatures, perhaps a desert, where thirsty people, say soldiers, could drink large amounts of them everyday. Some people might go as far as to say that these soldiers could experience long term effects from such exposure, and may have symptoms that replicate those of methanol or formaldehyde poisoning.

Strangely enough, Gulf War Syndrome (GWS) may have symptoms very similar to those seen in cases of methanol or formaldehyde poisoning. In fact "most symptoms of Gulf War Illness are similar to Chronic Fatigue Syndrome and/or Fibromyalgia."[122]

---

[120] Lohmann, K. Prohl, A. Schwarz, E. "Multiple chemical sensitivity disorder in patients with neurotoxic illnesses." **Gesundheitswesen** 1996 Jun;58(6):322-31.

[121] Smith, JD. Terpening, CM. Schmidt, SO. Gums, JG. "Relief of fibromyalgia symptoms following discontinuation of dietary excitotoxins." **Ann Pharmacother** 2001 Jun;35(6):702-6.

[122] Hannan, KL. Berg, DE. Baumzweiger, W. Harrison, HH. Berg, LH. Ramirez, R. Nichols, D. "Activation of the coagulation system in Gulf War Illness: a potential pathophysiologic link with chronic fatigue syndrome. A laboratory approach to diagnosis." **Blood Coagul Fibrinolysis** 2000 Oct;11(7):673-8.

Scientists studying victims of Gulf War Syndrome say that their symptomolagy "generally manifests as a set of nonspecific complaints with emphasis on central nervous system impairment."[123] Central nervous system impairment, where have we seen that before? That's what the American Academy of toxicology says happens when the body gets too much methanol. Thanks to the Nutrasweet Corporate Website, we know that Aspartame breaks down into methanol in the body. Could there be a link?

With the new influx of funding for the study and research of Gulf War Syndrome, perhaps some money could be set aside to test a hypothesis that examines the long term effect of heated soda containing Nutrasweet on the human body.

It would be rather disappointing if there was a connection between Aspartame and Gulf War Syndrome, for the simple reason that the Donald who pushed the approval of it through the FDA is now the Secretary of Defense: Donald Rumsfeld. Could he have poisoned the soldiers that now serve him?

Stepping away from conjecture to hard science, we can find another very interesting phenomenon: Aspartame can take on the same excitoxic qualities as Glutamate. Aspartic Acid (one of the amino acids in Aspartame) can affect the same neurons in the body that Glutamate does. It can even increase epileptic activity in children.[124]

Phenylalanine is the other amino acid that Aspartame breaks down into when digested. People with the genetically inherited syndrome, phenylketonuria, cannot properly metabolize this amino acid. For these people, Aspartame is a toxic substance. Pregnant mothers who have this condition and ingest Aspartame during

[123] Bunegin, L. Mitzel, HC. Miller, CS. Gelineau, JF. Tolstykh, GP. "Cognitive performance and cerebrohemodynamics associated with the Persian Gulf Syndrome." **Toxicol Ind Health** 2001 May;17(4):128-37.

[124] Camfield, PR. Camfield, CS. Dooley, JM. Gordon, K. Jollymore, S. Weaver, DF. "Aspartame exacerbates EEG spike-wave discharge in children with generalized absence epilepsy: a double-blind controlled study." **Neurology** 1992 May;42(5):1000-3.

pregnancy have a 93% chance of their baby becoming mentally retarded, and a 72% chance that their baby will be born with a substantially smaller brain.[125] If Aspartame can cause birth defects such as these, is it really a healthy alternative to sugar?

Perhaps the scientists of the companies who produced Nutrasweet know more about its questionable safety than they are saying.

G.D. Searle, 4 years after marketing Aspartame, was sold with the help of Donald Rumsfeld to Monsanto Company in 1985. In December of 1999 Monsanto announced it was merging with Pharmacia & Upjohn. On March 23rd, 2000 both company's shareholders voted to approve the merger. The merger was to take place on March 31st. But on March 27th, four days after the shareholders voted to approve the merger and four days before the company's merger, Monsanto approved the sale of its Aspartame interests. It sold its international interests to Ajinomoto Corporation (the MSG giant) for 67 million, and its American Nutrasweet Company to J.W. Childs Equity Partners II, L.P for $440 million in cash.[126] Why would a company divest itself of a half billion dollars in corporate value just days before a merger? Perhaps Pharmacia and Upjohn did not want Nutrasweet on their hands. As it stands now, J.W. Childs Equity Partners II, L.P, are the new owners of Nutrasweet. J. W. Childs is a private investment firm. The true financiers who backed their purchase of Nutrasweet hide behind a veil of anonymity, possibly protecting themselves from liability issues that could develop if Nutrasweet were found to be toxic.

For me to put something in my children's mouths, I want to know that the company that created a product stands behind the product 100%. With all the corporate restructuring surrounding Aspartame, who knows where the blame for Aspartame's ills would go.

---

[125] Hanley, WB. Clarke, JT. Schoonheyt, W. "Maternal phenylketonuria (PKU)--a review." **Clin Biochem** 1987 Jun;20(3):149-56.

[126] www.monsanto.com.

I also want to know that the product I feed to my children was thoroughly tested and wasn't rushed through the FDA approval process by people interested more in profits and politics than the safety of the nation.

Aspartame has its own promotional association called the Calorie Control Council. Just like the Glutamate Association, their membership is made up of manufacturers and suppliers of artificial sweeteners and products. Just like the Glutamate Association, their membership list is private, though the Calorie Control Council does offer a "select list of companies and products serving health-conscious consumers."[127] Not surprisingly, Ajinomoto Corporation and the Nutrasweet Company are on this list. The mission statements of these two unrelated associations are so similar, it looks like they copied them from each other.

Calorie Control Council:

The Council seeks to provide an effective channel of communication among its members, the public and government officials, and to assure that scientific, medical and other pertinent research and information is developed and made available to all interested parties. http://www.caloriecontrol.org/aboutCCC.html

Glutamate Association

The Glutamate Association seeks to provide an effective channel of communication among its members, the public, the media, the scientific community, food professionals and government officials about the use and safety of Glutamates. The Association also seeks to assure that relevant research and information on the safety and efficacy of MSG are made available to all interested parties. http://www.msgfacts.com/aboutus.html

Two unrelated organizations, sharing almost exactly the same mission statements in the same order, seem strangely suspect.

---

[127] *www.caloriecontrol.org*

Their mission: to make sure that "pertinent" or "relevant" information are made available? How do they decide what is pertinent or relevant. Perhaps only things that protect their profit margin are considered pertinent and relevant. These two organizations try to make propaganda sound like an altruistic endeavor.

The whole purpose of these associations' existence is to promote their products for their own profit. This is further shown by the fact that the Calorie Control Council is fronted by the Kellen company, a for profit company that specializes in providing executive directing and management to 47 such associations representing over 5000 companies. Their list of clients includes both the International Food Additives Council, and International Glutamate Technical Committee.

Kellen Company's purpose to represent the companies in the associations they manage is no secret. They advertise it on their Website 'www.assnhq.com' to sell their services.

Kellen Company states:

"Our aggressive leadership and respected relationships with Congress, regulatory agencies, the media, health and scientific groups and other opinion leaders significantly benefit our clients." They boast that their *"professionals have extensive experience in government affairs, working with FDA, USDA, EPA, OSHA, CPSC, FTC, DOT and other federal and related state agencies on a variety of issues"* and that with these agencies their *"company is respected for its factual, scientifically based approach."* [128]

Here I thought that all those government organizations were on the side of the consumer.

Worst of all, the Kellen Company declares that they *"impact (and have drafted) regulations and legislation now in place affecting the*

---

[128] www.assnhq.com

industries we represent."[129] Here I thought that in the democratic country of America, it is the elected representatives that create regulations and legislation.

The Kellen Company, one of the largest association representation companies in America, on the bankroll of 5000 companies, advertises what believers in democracy have always feared: they, a partisan, corporate controlled entity, impact on and even draft the regulations and laws that control the industries they represent.

It seems that in America, criminals can write their own laws.

Have a toxic pollutant you want to get rid of? Have the Public Health Service put it in the nations water supply.

Have a brain-manipulating drug that makes people eat more? Get the FDA to declare it safe for use in uncontrolled quantities.

Have a patented sweetener that can cause brain tumors? Have some questionable politicians ram it through the approval process.

Isn't America great?

It sure is for corporations.

All is not lost, we consumers have a watchdog looking out for our interests. It's called the Center for Food Safety and Applied Nutrition (CFSAN). This is a division of the FDA whose primary function is consumer protection. Finally we have hope. The CFSAN has an Adverse Reaction Monitoring System (ARMS), to collect data on consumers contacting them to complain about problems they have with food additives. The director, J. Levitt, states that the ARMS was created in 1985 to collect data on adverse reactions to Aspartame and MSG. He pointed this fact out to the Committee on Government Reform on May 27th, 1999.

---

[129] www.assnhq.com

Surely the data collected by the ARMS would prompt the Center for Food Safety and Applied Nutrition to reexamine the safety of MSG and Aspartame. This was not to be. In 1999, the Adverse Reaction Monitoring System was cancelled. A letter from J. Levitt was written on August 29, 2002 to say the ARMS centralized data collection was scrapped in 1999. The letter was strangely distressing, it was addressed to "Stakeholders," and at the end of the letter asked the "trade associations" to forward the letter to their members. References to the consumer public were nowhere to be found.

Is the FDA's primary function not consumer protection? Was not the Adverse Reaction Monitoring System put in place to listen to the concerns of the consumer? Shouldn't the public, not the trade associations, be the only stakeholders the FDA should answer to?

I dug deeper into the inner workings of the CFSAN and was disappointed by what I found.

In the CFSAN Priority Setting meeting on June 24th and 25th, 1998 there was an amazing representation of corporate associations.

In attendance were the American Frozen Food Institute, the Grocery Manufacturers of America, the Enzyme Technical Association (Ajinomoto is a member), the Calorie Control Council, (Ajinomoto is a member of this too), The Association for Dressings and Sauces, (members like Kraft and once again, Ajinomoto), as well as the Alliance of Food Additive Producers (including members like Monsonto, Frito-Lay, Kraft, and Campbells).

Just to make sure they got their point abundantly clear, Kraft sent a direct representative as well.

Most of these companies were at the Priorities Meeting to request that the process to make a food ingredient Generally Recognized as Safe (GRAS) easier for the manufacturer. The International Hydrolyzed Protein Council was also at the meeting demanding that the FDA not require them to label HVP as Glutamate on products.

The meeting wasn't all one sided, one consumer group was represented there. Dr. Jacobson, from the Center for Science in the Public Interest, tried to hold his own against the wolves. He asked the CFSAN to "promptly approve well-founded health claims that would promote an overall healthier diet." Maybe he meant the research proving the danger of Aspartame and MSG. He outlined the "need for greater authority to protect the public from unsafe and misleadingly labeled products." He asked that the FDA tighten its poorly run approval process, and urged them to carefully scrutinize substances that already had GRAS status.

It is five years later and none of his requests have come to pass. The well-represented associations fared much better. 1998 was a good year for Procter and Gamble and Frito-Lay. Olestra, the 'no-fat' fat alternative introduced in 1996 and described by Dr. Jacobson as "the most complained about food additive in history" got a clean bill of health from the FDA, despite the frequent side effects of gastrointestinal upset. After all, why should the FDA protect the consumer when they can protect the profiteering manufacturer? Once they start banning every artificial ingredient that makes some people sick they'd end up following their primary directive of protecting the consumer. Where is the profit in that?

Sadly, it seems that J. Levitt and his team at CFSAN spend more time listening to the product associations than they did to the consumers they are supposed to protect.

Now before Canadians reading this start snickering at the bureaucratic folly rampant both in the FDA and the American legislative process, you had better look in your own backyard. The Center for Science in the Public Interest (CSPI) has offices in Canada too and there the prognosis doesn't look much better.

In an article titled Canadian Food Information Council: Wolf in Sheep's Clothing, Bill Jeffery of the CSPI states that the Canadian Food Information Council (CFIC) which influences public and government opinion, is secretly funded by Monsonto, Kraft, Procter and Gamble (makers of toxic fluoridated toothpaste and

Olestra), and many other giant food and chemical manufacturers. The CFIC "has dismissed concerns about the safety of Monosodium Glutamate (MSG), caffeine, artificial sweeteners, irradiation, and other controversial food additives and processes."[130]

Canada's government has ended up being a sad reflection of what happens in Washington. Why is it that Canadians get angry when they are referred to as the 51st state? Their politicians certainly act like it is.

---

130 Jeffery, Bill. 'Canadian Food Information Council: Wolf in Sheep's Clothing.' May 23rd, 2000.

Mad Cow: Coming Soon to a Grill Near You?

Newspapers, radio, and television stations across the country blasted the news: Canada has its first Mad Cow.

The Canadian government leapt into action. Like a well-oiled censorship machine it gave only the smallest amount of information to the media and the Canadian people. After all, they wouldn't want a panic situation like the one in Britain that almost wiped out the entire beef industry there.

People are not the only ones who suffer the affects of unnatural additives in their food supply. The animals that we depend on for food, and in turn depend on us to feed them, are also at risk of human engineered food additives. Just as MSG and Aspartame can be dangerous to humans, ingredients in the diets of the cattle, sheep, pigs, and chickens can be harmful to them.

It was these additives that caused the Mad Cow epidemic in Great Britain, leading to the infection and destruction of almost a million cattle and the tragic death of 129 people.

Mad Cow disease is known medically as bovine spongiform encephalopathy (BSE). It is a disease that can pass between species and is fatal in 100% of its cases. Strains of transmissible spongiform encephalopathy(TSE) have been found to kill sheep, deer, elk, mice, cattle, chimpanzees, domestic house cats and even humans.

In 1986, the first case of Mad Cow disease appeared in Great Britain. The British government learned that the cause of the disease was directly linked to the nutritional additives fed to their livestock. For years farmers had been feeding their cattle with feed made from ground up cattle meat and bones.

The farmers had turned their grass-eating cows into cannibals.

What would make farmers turn this gentle animal into a carnivorous beast?

Profit.

Decades ago, pharmaceutical giants like Monsanto created bovine growth hormones that when given to cattle had amazing results. Dairy cows would produce substantially more milk, and butcher cattle would grow meat faster and in greater amounts.

The downside of this diet was that it required the cattle to be fed larger amounts of protein then they could get in the standard farm diet. Feed suppliers came to the answer with a product referred to as by-pass protein. This supplement has large amounts of protein in it. While plant based protein supplements are available, the ones made from animal products are usually cheaper.

Farmers gravitated to the cheaper feed and soon feeding dead cows to live cows became a standard process.

In 1988, the government of the U.K. declared a ban on this cannibalistic practice, and hoped that this would end the feared epidemic. The action seems to have helped, but it was too little too late.

By the year 2002, mad cow disease had spread to 181, 376 cattle.

Almost a million head of cattle had to be destroyed to stop the contagion.

Throughout the epidemic, the government swore that Mad Cow disease could not be transmitted to humans through the eating of beef. Prime Minister John Major promoted the safety of beef by eating steak on national television.

The British population believed him, until the first human died in 1996 from the horrific disease. The human strain of transmissible spongiform encephalopathy is referred to as variant Creutzfeldt-Jakob disease (vCJD).

Variant Creutzfeldt-Jakob disease is a terrible degenerative disease that begins with the victims behaving in a depressed or paranoid way. They become progressively demented, followed by loss of bodily control, coma, and death. According to the World Health Organization, 129 people have died in the U.K. from vCJD contracted from food contaminated with Mad Cow disease.[131] The disease seems to strike young people, with teenagers and young adults making up the majority of the victims.

The first human death from eating contaminated beef appeared in 1996, ten years after the first case of Mad Cow, and 8 years after the government of the U.K. banned the exercise of feeding ground up cows to cattle.

The governments of Canada and United States have watched the disaster across the ocean, but have been slow in learning from Britain's mistakes. Bovine growth hormones have also been used heavily in here, and our cattle have been fed ground up cows for years. Though this disgusting practice was banned in Great Britain in 1988, the cattle in Canada and the U.S. continued to dine on their brothers, sisters, parents and even offspring until 1997. Only in 1997, once it was confirmed that Mad Cow disease could kill

---

[131] World Health Organization, 'Bovine Spongiform Encephalopathy', **WHO Fact Sheet** no.113 November 2000.

people, did these governments adopt policies to stop the practice that creates the mad cow disease.

In Britain it was a case of too little too late. What will be the case here?

The U.S. and Canada have stopped the feeding of cows to cattle, but they can still be fed meat and bone meal from pigs, horses, and chickens. Cattle, whose digestive systems are designed to live on plant matter, are still on a carnivorous diet. The governments overlook a disastrous loophole: Diseased cows can be fed to chickens; ground up chickens can be fed back to cows. The agent that causes Mad Cow disease can collect in chickens, and then be fed back to the cows. Thus the virus that causes Mad Cow can still find its way back into the cow feed it was banned from.

In many rendering plants, the new regulation to stop putting cow meat into cow feed has not been followed. In United States between 1998 and 2000, "FDA and state inspectors visited 9,184 rendering firms to increase awareness of the BSE regulation only to find that 1,688 of the firms were not aware of the new regulation."[132] Even after the federally mandated ban, almost 20 percent of rendering plants inspected were still bagging cattle meat as cow feed. How confident can we be in the government's attempts to avoid a mad cow epidemic?

The Canadian government has been very careful in the information that they pass on to the media. Included in this selective censorship is any detailed information regarding the high infection risk of Mad Cow disease.

Noted scientist Stanley Prusiner developed the primary theory behind the cause of spongiform encephalopathy in the 1980's. Prusiner discovered a protein strain that he named 'prion.'

---

[132] Hileman, B. 'The mad disease has many forms.' **Chemical and Engineering News.** Vol 79 - 15 pp.24-30.

Prions (pronounced pree-on) are found to occur in mammals. The problem occurs when a defective prion is introduced in the body and programs the host DNA to change the existing prions into mutant ones. These mutant prion molecules seem to affect the brain matter of the host, causing sponge like holes to appear.

Prions do not behave like standard viruses. They are strands of amino acids that do not have DNA, and are not even alive. As such they are unable to be killed by sterilization, irradiation, or even heating to 600 degrees Fahrenheit.

A great deal of research supports Prusiner's theory. Unfortunately, the research also proved his theory that infectious prions are almost impossible to destroy. Electrodes that had been used on the brain of a woman with CJD transferred the disease to two other humans that they were later used on. After two years, three cleanings and repeated sterilization with ethanol and formaldehyde, the electrodes were implanted into the brain of a chimpanzee. The chimpanzee contracted CJD and died.[133]

Most scientists scoffed at Prusiner's theory, but in 1996, his research on prions won him the Nobel Prize. Now his theory is regarded as the foremost scientific explanation for the transmission of this deadly disease.

The World Health Organization recognizes Prusiner's research, and reports that the only effective way to completely stop the risk of infection from BSE contaminated objects is to incinerate them. Standard methods of chemical disinfection and heat sterilization are not fully effective at reducing the prions ability to infect other life forms.[134]

Agriculture Canada claimed that the contaminated cow first discovered in January 2003 in Alberta did not present a threat to

---

[133] Gibbs, CJ Jr. Asher, DM. Kobrine, A. Amyx, HL. Sulima, MP. Gajdusek, DC. 'Transmission of Creutzfeldt-Jakob disease to a chimpanzee by electrodes contaminated during neurosurgery.' **J Neurol Neurosurg Psychiatry** 1994 Jun;57(6):757-8.

[134] World Health Organization, 'WHO infection control guidelines for transmissible spongiform encephalopathy.' Geneva Switzerland, March 1999, Page 13.

the food supply. The inspector at the slaughterhouse that discovered the sickly cow marked it unfit for human consumption. The cow was disemboweled using the same equipment that afterwards cut up cattle destined for Canadian dinner plates. Its organs were spread across an examining table. The head was severed from the body and sent to a government site to be tested. The inspector determined that the meat was unfit for human consumption and sent it to a rendering plant.

Three months later, testing proved that the cow was infected with the Mad Cow prion. Three months had gone by during which an unidentified number of cows were cut up using the same implements that butchered the infected cow. If hospital sterilization methods cannot disinfect contaminated implements, what chance do the wash down procedures at a slaughterhouse have?

The prions left at the slaughterhouse are not the only ones consumers should worry about. The carcass of the infected cow was sent to a rendering plant, where the meat and bones were ground up to make animal feed and pet food, or boiled to make gelatin. The bags of feed were sold to farmers, to be fed to pigs and chickens. It is believed that neither pigs nor chickens are susceptible to the mutant prion disorder, but there is no evidence that the infective mad cow agent does not remain dormant in the tissues of either animal. From there it could be fed to humans, or end up in feed served back to cattle.

Unfortunately, the pet food situation is much more frightening. According to an FDA report dated May 26th, 2003, the government of Canada informed them that its first Mad Cow could have been rendered into dry dog food and sold to the American market under the brand name Pet Pantry of America. Since the cow was turned into pet food in February, the bags of food could have already been sold and fed to dogs. The FDA report goes on to say that dogs do not contract bovine spongiform encephalopathy and says that there's no evidence that dogs can transmit it to humans.[135] The

---

[135] U.S. Food and Drug Administration. 'FDA BSE Update - Pet Food from Canadian Manufacturer.' FDA Statement May 26, 2003.

FDA however, is terribly short on details. The warning does not inform the consumer that human handling of the dry dog food could transmit the prion contaminant to humans. They completely avoid telling people who have a dog and cat in the house that cats have proven to be susceptible to infection from BSE prions, and that many domestic cats in the United Kingdom have died from the disease. Prions themselves are not destroyed when they pass through a dog's digestive system, so dog food made from the Mad Cow may end up covering someone's lawn with prion-infected landmines.

Long after Canada's first Mad Cow was found, the byproducts of its demise are haunting consumers across North America.

The prions that cause transmissible spongiform encephalopathy tend to collect in the brain, spinal column, nerve tissue, bones and lymphatic system of the cow. This news is what the government points at to suggest that eating beef is safe. If they really believe that prions aren't found anywhere else in cattle's infected bodies, why is the Canadian Blood Service that collects and supplies the nation with blood refusing to except blood donations from anyone who has spent more than 3 months in Great Britain since 1980. Is blood and the meat that it's in really that safe? The FDA even stated in 1996 that blood donations should no longer be taken from those who have come from the United Kingdom. In 1999 they revised this warning to include anyone who may have used bovine insulin produced from there.[136] So what aren't these agencies telling us?

When Shirley McClellan, Alberta's minister of agriculture mimicked Britain's Prime Minister by posing for the photo-op of her eating a juicy steak, was it well done or rare? Not that it matters; cooking can't destroy prions.

---

[136] U.S. Food and Drug Administration. 'Revised Preventive Measures to Reduce the Possible Risk of Transmission of Creutzfeldt-Jakob Disease (CJD) and Variant Creutzfeldt-Jakob Disease (vCJD) by Blood and Blood Products.' January 2002.

Rendering plants, like the one that Canada's first mad cow went to, boil up the connective tissues and bones to create gelatin. This gelatin is then sold to many processing companies. Gelatin is one of the 650 products made from cattle for human use.[137] Gelatin is especially popular in candy, jello and marshmallows, all of which are highly desired by children.

The WHO states that substances like "gelatin are considered safe if prepared by a manufacturing process which has been shown experimentally to inactivate the transmissible agent."[138] Strangely enough, the only process that the WHO states can completely inactivate prions is incineration. The processes that produce gelatin do not come close to such temperature extremes.

The by-products of rendering plants are not just used in food. They are also found in cosmetics, drugs, vaccines, insulin, even the collagen that women have injected into their faces for beauty's sake. Both collagen[139] and gelatin[140] have been considered possible sources for mad cow transmission to humans.

Rendering plants are a weak link in the nations food supply. They are the final destination for the chickens, pigs, deer and cattle that are not fit for human consumption. One city in United States was even caught sending euthanized dogs and cats from their animal control building to a rendering plant to be added to the mix.[141] Imagine feeding that to your dog or cat.

We count on these rendering plants for much of the protein feed supplements that go to feed the chickens, pigs, and cattle that we

[137] Rampton, S. Stauber, J. Mad Cow U.S.A. Common Courage Press, 1997. Page 210.

[138] World Health Organization, 'Bovine Spongiform Encephalopathy.' **WHO Fact Sheet** No. 113, November 2002.

[139] Lupi, O. 'Prions in dermatology.' **J Am Acad Dermatol** 2002 May;46(5):790-3.

[140] Schrieber, R. Seybold, U. "Gelatine production, the six steps to maximum safety.' **Dev Biol Stand** 1993;80:195-8.

[141] Allman, J. 'Mayor: Pets from city pound will not go to plant' KMOV Channel 4 News, St. Louis. Dec 14th, 2001.

consume on a daily basis. Does it give us confidence knowing that most of the animals used at these plants were too diseased or unhealthy to feed us directly? The cattle that are sent to these plants are referred to as 'downer cows' meaning they do not have the strength to stand up again once they have lain down. Many of these cows are sent for rendering without any tests to see what their ailment was. If the cow in Canada had not been suffering from pneumonia-like symptoms, and had its brain sent for further testing, what would have happened? How many infected cows have passed through undetected already?

Every week in Canada, over 90 million pounds of cattle that have died of 'natural causes' are rendered[142] into hundreds of products for use all over North America. Of these cattle, only the smallest percentage is tested to see if they died from Mad Cow disease.

With bovine spongiform encephalopathy (BSE), it is entirely possible that infected cattle might go to slaughter before any symptoms of the disease are observed. If this were the case, how much of the cattle meat and by-products would find their way to our tables, cosmetics, and medicine cabinets?

We have much to learn from the United Kingdom's mistakes. Recently it was reported that the U.K. Food Standards Agency discovered that British consumers ate millions of hamburgers containing material that was potentially infected with BSE. The ground beef in question contained mechanically removed meat from the spines of cattle. Most of this meat was sent to school and institutional cafeterias.[143] The spinal column and nerve tissues are some of the body parts considered by the World Health Organization to be the most infectious.

The government needs to be more honest with consumers about the full ramifications of a Mad Cow epidemic. Britain kept its people in the dark, promoting the safety of eating beef in spite of the

---

[142] CBC News Online: 'Canadian farmers face dead cattle pile up.' May, 2003.

[143] Meikle, J. 'BSE meat went into millions of burgers.' **The Guardian**, London, England. Oct. 11th, 2002.

disease. 129 people died because of their propaganda, how many more will?

Chronic Wasting Disease

Cattle aren't the only carriers of transmissible spongiform encephalopathy (TSE). United States and Canada are quietly suffering from an epidemic of 'Mad Deer.'

When mutant prions infect deer the result is called Chronic Wasting Disease (CWD). Infected deer become listless, walk irregularly, and finally die from irreversible weight loss. First discovered in Colorado in 1967, this disease has now spread to encompass deer herds in Wyoming, Nebraska, Saskatchewan, and even Alberta.

In Alberta the disease has struck both deer and elk. Over 15,000 of these animals are killed each year in Alberta alone. Rendering plants will no longer process their carcasses due to chance of prion infection. Their bodies are ending up in the landfills and ditches all over Alberta.[144]

As these bodies decompose, the infective prions within them may make their way into the soil and ground water. CWD has been found to infect deer simply from being present on the ground the deer graze on.[145]

Tragically, CWD is transmissible between species. It has been discovered that young cattle injected with CWD from deer have developed the disease and when autopsied had mutant prions in

---

[144] Duckworth, B. 'Safe carcass disposal method studied.' **The Western Producer,** Saskatoon, May 21st, 2003.

[145] Hileman, B. 'The mad disease has many forms.' **Chemical and Engineering News.** Volume 79 Number 15 pp.24-30.

their brain matter.[146]   With CWD infecting deer in areas heavily populated by cattle, how long will it be before the disease creates an epidemic in the species used for the human food supply?

The prion threat is real, and unless serious precautions are taken, America may see the same devastation that the U.K did, not only to its cattle, but to its people as well.

---

[146] Hamir, AN. Cutlip, RC. Miller, JM. Williams, ES. Stack, MJ. Miller, MW. O'Rourke, KI. Chaplin, MJ. 'Preliminary findings on the experimental transmission of chronic wasting disease agent of mule deer to cattle.' **J Vet Diagn Invest** 2001 Jan;13(1):91-6.

The Overlooked, Undercooked, Threat

In the United Kingdom, Mad Cow disease infected almost 200,000 cows. It almost destroyed the beef industry of the entire country. It is a disease that is feared by both governments of United States and Canada.

There is a disease in America, however, that poses an even greater threat then Mad Cow disease.

In the time that it took for a strain of Mad Cow disease to kill 129 people in the United Kingdom, an overlooked contaminant in the American food supply killed over 400 people.

The Center for Disease Control estimates that in United States, this disease kills 61 people, and sickens 73,000 men, women and children each year.

This disease transmits easily between people; especially family members and child care workers.

This disease can contaminate drinking water, rivers, lakes and swimming pools.

This disease causes severe and even bloody diarrhea. It can lead to kidney failure. In fact, it is the number one cause of kidney failure in children.

There is no known cure or treatment for this disease.

What is the primary cause of this frightening disease?

Beef.

Undercooked, ground beef.[147]

The beef and dairy cow carries the bacteria that causes far more death and illness than almost any other food born illness in America.

Escherichia coli O157:H7 is the bacteria's name. There are many strains of bacteria commonly referred to as E. Coli. This one, however, is toxic to humans.

Unlike the deadly prion, this E. Coli strain doesn't harm the animal it was created in. The cattle that carry it remain healthy. They quietly are stripped of their milk, or head off to the slaughterhouse to be killed for their meat. Pasteurization supposedly kills the E. Coli present in milk, but raw meat is not processed that way. It is shipped off to the supermarket or restaurant with the dangerous E. Coli still living within it.

E. Coli food poisoning was first diagnosed in 1982, when many people suffered bloody diarrhea after eating hamburgers.

The case of the outbreak was linked to a bacteria only found to exist in the intestinal system in cattle. Since its first discovery, this strain of E. Coli has caused hundreds of death, and possibly millions of illnesses in North America alone.

---

[147] Center for Disease Control. 'Escherichia coli O157:H7 Frequently Asked Questions' **Division of Bacterial and Mycotic Diseases**. www.cdc.gov.

Children are the hardest hit by this sickness. The bacteria destroy their red blood cells, leading to kidney failure. This disorder is called hemolytic uremic syndrome. The Center for Disease Control states that of the children that get E. Coli poisoning, 2-7 percent will develop this deadly disorder. The disorder is common enough to make E. Coli poisoning the number one cause of kidney failure in America's children.

The primary way people contract E. Coli poisoning is through eating improperly cooked hamburgers or unpasteurized milk. Hamburger improperly stored can contaminate work surfaces in kitchens, restaurants and grocery stores. Fruits and vegetables that are eaten raw can pick up the contamination from the raw meat residues. How often have you visited the grocery store, and seen hamburger packages drip their blood onto the check out conveyor belt. That blood may have dripped in the cart where you have set your toddler, or been smeared on the cart handle. E. Coli germs can remain infective for up to twenty weeks.[148] Without thorough cooking or a proper disinfecting with bleach. E. Coli germs from hamburger could contaminate you, your food, and your children. E. Coli bacteria are even resistant to normal refrigeration and freezing. Contaminated items purchased today could harm you months from now.

In humans, toxic cattle E. Coli remains in the digestive system for 5-10 days. They leave the body through the stool. This stool is then an infective agent. Healthcare and childcare workers are especially at risk to secondary infection from the bacteria. These bacteria are especially virulent in water.

When the E. Coli bacteria are flushed with the stool into the public waste, they can remain toxic unless properly treated at a waste facility. Unfortunately, many populations are without proper treatment facilities. Halifax is the thriving capital of Nova Scotia with over 360,000 inhabitants. Despite its wealth as a successful

---

[148] Health Canada, 'An outbreak of escherichia *coli* O157:H7 infection associated with unpasteurized non commercial, custom-pressed apple cider' **Canada Communicable Disease Report.** July 1999. Vol 25-13.

city, "four-fifths of Halifax's industrial and municipal sewage is pumped directly into the harbour."[149] Without proper treatment, E. Coli bacteria can remain a deadly infective agent, ready to spread to an unsuspecting public.

Halifax is not the only metropolitan area that does not practice safe sewage treatment methods, cities all around the shores of Lake Ontario pumped enough raw sewage in it to not only destroy the lake but also make it dangerous to swim in.

The Great Lakes are interconnected; it is hard to pollute one without affecting the others. Canada and United States take pride in having a huge supply of fresh water to draw on, and cities on both sides of the border use these lakes as their drinking water supply. But just how fresh is this water?

Citizens of Walkerton, Ontario were happy to go about their daily lives, trusting that the government was providing them with safe drinking water.

In May of 2000, their trust was shattered, and may never again return.

One spring day in 2000 a farmer climbed on his tractor and proceeded to spread cattle manure on a field. This a common practice in agricultural areas and the farmer spread it following the government standards.

Unfortunately, around the 12th of May, the manure the farmer had spread seeped into one of the supply wells for the city of Walkerton. Workers at the Walkerton public utilities did not act quickly on tests that showed E. Coli was in the drinking water. They did not add the appropriate level of chlorine to kill the bacteria. Not until the 21st of May, nine days after the contamination occurred, did the local government authorities warn the public of the danger. In that time the men, women and children

[149] McMahon, F. 'Halifax's political sewage problem.' **National Post**. July 13th, 1999.

of Walkerton ingested enough toxic E. Coli from cattle manure to poison 2,300 residents and kill seven.

Many of the children who survived the outbreak developed hemolytic uremic syndrome, damaging their kidneys permanently. The CDC details the long-term effects:

> *About one-third of persons with hemolytic uremic syndrome have abnormal kidney function many years later, and a few require long-term dialysis. Another 8% of persons with hemolytic uremic syndrome have other lifelong complications, such as high blood pressure, seizures, blindness, paralysis, and the effects of having part of their bowel removed.*[150]

Long-term illness.

That could be Walkerton's price for living near fields that cattle manure gets spread on. The farmer who caused the E. Coli infestation was not considered at fault. Government guidelines protected him. What guidelines protected the residents of Walkerton?

Public water systems are available in most cities and towns in the United States and Canada. The people who live in villages and rural areas use water from private wells. In many cases, the fields the farmers spread their cow manure on are only a short distance away from the wells that their neighbors drink from. If run-off from neighboring fields can contaminate a government monitored public water supply, what can they do to well water?

To those of you who do not have the safety of public water treatment (Walkerton residents could argue this), do you know what is going into your drinking water?

---

[150] Center for Disease Control. 'Escherichia coli O157:H7 Frequently Asked Questions' **Division of Bacterial and Mycotic Diseases**. www.cdc.gov.

Even if your water is safe, E. Coli from cattle is prevalent in foods that our children eat everyday. Thousands of tonnes of ground beef are served to our children in cafeterias, fast food restaurants, and at home.

Cattle that carry harmful E. Coli bacteria are outwardly healthy. They show no visible signs of the infection. Meat inspectors do not test for the presence of E. Coli before allowing the beef into the human food supply. Since its discovery in 1982, millions of people have taken ill from its presence in hamburgers. Lawsuits of restaurant chains such as Jack in the Box that have distributed E. Coli infected burgers, are proof of the dangers that threaten consumers.

Eric Schlosser, author of the New York Times best-selling book *Fast Food Nation*, has made himself an authority on the restaurant industry in the United States. In an article called 'Bad Meat' written for the publication: *The Nation*, Schlosser outlines the incredible danger of E. Coli infection, and the federal governments lack of control.

Schlosser points out that the USDA no longer has the ability to stop meatpacking plants from distributing contaminated beef. Company employees now do the meat inspection at their own processing plants. USDA inspectors can only do random tests for E. Coli bacteria at wholesale and retail locations. By the time the inspectors locate any tainted meat, consumers may already have purchased it.

To show the enormous power that the meat industry has over the government, Schlosser details a case where the USDA shut down a Texas company, Supreme Meat Processors, one of the largest suppliers of meat to the National School Lunch Program. The USDA repeatedly found salmonella, a bacteria that sickens over a million Americans each year, in the Supreme Meat Processor's meat products. The USDA closed down the plant in November of 1999. With the help of the meat packing industry, Supreme Meat Processors sued the federal government and won. They went on to influence the government into overturning salmonella limitations in beef products. Now it is legal in the USA to sell beef that is thoroughly contaminated with salmonella to all US citizens, including the young ones that use the National School Lunch Program.

Schlosser points out that federal law does not even require a meat processing plant to keep a list of suppliers they ship to. The USDA can't even track an infected meat shipment from the source to the restaurants or stores it supplies.[151]

This does not bode well for the protection of people from Mad Cow when it does rear its head in the USA. How do we know it hasn't already? Since meat safety inspection is now in the hands of the company that slaughters the beef, how do we know that they haven't hidden any dangerous findings? What profitable company wants to be the first to cry Mad Cow?

With the USDA intimidated by the meat suppliers, how safe do you feel putting that hamburger in your child's mouth? Schlosser states that as long as the USDA wears two hats, that of meat inspector and that of promoter of American meat consumption, the consumer will never be properly protected.

Avoiding hamburger altogether is no guarantee that you and your family won't get E. Coli poisoning from cattle. Dairy cows also transmit the toxin in their milk. The Center for Disease Control would have you believe that only unpasteurized milk can carry risk of E. Coli poisoning, but this is not accurate.

On June 1st, 2000, a USDA inspection of Breakstone small curd cottage cheese showed that the product contained toxic E. Coli bacteria. Cottage cheese is most often eaten cold, and the E. Coli could have led to a considerable outbreak of disease. Kraft, the parent company, was quick to voluntarily recall the product, which had already been sold to consumers in stores in various locations. I do not know how Kraft or the FDA hoped to reach all the people who bought their product. Very few of these recalls get the media

---

[151] Schlosser, E. 'Bad Meat.' **The Nation.** August 29, 2002.

attention needed to thoroughly protect the population. In fact, the FDA has so many recalls on a regular basis that it could justify its own television and radio station just to announce them all.

How did E. Coli get into pasteurized cottage cheese? The FDA never bothered to find out. They were content with the fact that Kraft recalled the items. What would have happened if a USDA inspector had not made an onsite visit to the factory? The infected batch sent out for consumption had already passed the company quality inspection unit, and was on store shelves when the USDA inspector made the E. Coli discovery and ask for the June recall.

When a company is left to inspect its own products for the consumer's safety, the conflict of interest creates considerable room for deliberate error. The letter from the FDA to the Chief Executive Officer of Colgate-Palmolive (referred to on page 28) regarding tainted toothpaste made this perfectly clear.

There are not enough FDA inspectors to ensure the public's safety. Kraft claims to be sincerely interested in protecting the public from health risks. Considering that Kraft is owned by Philip Morris, tobacco giant whose products have caused countless deaths due to cancer, how interested in protecting the public health could they be?

There remains no answer as to how the dangerous E. Coli bacteria from dairy cattle got into the Kraft food designed to be eaten without cooking. If it can happen in cottage cheese, E. Coli could contaminate sour cream, yogurt, cream and even milk. If no FDA inspectors were in the food plants to stop the dangerous contamination, our first warning would be the sight of our loved ones getting sick.

Mad Cow may be a serious threat to the food supply, but E. Coli from cattle already is. So far this simple bacteria, which meat packing plants will not let government inspectors test for, has killed more people in three years than Mad Cow has in ten.

The Antidotes

Fear not, there is hope. With enough of us waking from our sheep-like sleep we can make our voices heard. We can put an end to the poisoning that our children and ourselves suffer at the hands of profiteers and governments.

Whether the poison has been added to our water supply, heaped into our processed foods and drinks, or contaminating our meat supplies, we as consumers and parents, have a say in our health and safety.

Fluoride poisoning can be stopped.

The governments of United States and Canada must accept the scientific evidence and join the dozens of other countries that recognize the dangers of fluoride in the water supply.

The addition of fluoride to water should be banned. Industries pumping the toxin into our streams, rivers and lakes must immediately stop, and be held accountable for the pollution they have caused.

The dental community and companies that produce dental products should stop the use and promotion of fluoride. There are currently a number of toothpaste manufacturers that make non-fluoridated toothpaste which are sold at pharmacies, health food stores and the health food sections in some grocery stores.

Communities with naturally occurring fluoride in the water should avoid using it without the fluoride being filtered out. An in-home reverse osmosis unit can remove fluoride. Federal assistance should be made available to remove the fluoride from community wells. In 1931, both the American Dental Association and the United States Public Health service requested this action. 72 years late is better than never.

MSG and Aspartame can easily be removed from America's food supplies. The FDA, and Health Canada, simply by declaring that they are dangerous to human health, can immediately stop their addition to our foods. All current stocks of food items tainted with these neurotoxins can be recalled and sent back to their manufacturers. The people of United States and Canada do not need to be drugged into choosing one product over another, and they certainly don't want to be misled by a chemical alternative that is more damaging to the body than the sugar it is meant to replace.

Cattle that threaten us with toxic E. Coli bacteria or Mad Cow disease can be removed from the food chain.

The U. S. Food and Drug Agency (FDA) is currently promoting industries to use powerful irradiation at the processing plants to kill bacteria such as E. Coli. Though consumer groups quote a great deal of research showing the process is a danger to health, and suggesting that instead better care should be taken to raise healthy livestock, the FDA is pushing for the irradiation of foods to become widespread.

An article for the *FDA Consumer Magazine*, called *Irradiation: A Safe Measure for Safer Food*, written by the agency's staff, states that "Trade groups such as the National Meat Association, the Grocery Manufacturers of America, and the National Food Processors Association also support irradiation......with so many influential organizations backing irradiation......the stage is set for the process to pick up momentum, despite negative sentiments."[152]

It seems obvious whose side the U.S. Food and Drug Administration are on. Instead of taking E. Coli infected cattle from the food chain, they intend to submit our food to high levels of radiation. They have already authorized the use of food irradiation on fruits and vegetables, and not for the reason of killing bacteria or protecting the public. They approved its use to slow the aging of vegetables, so the grocery stores can keep them on the shelves longer. Does adding radiation to lettuce and strawberries help the consumer, or rather those geared to profit from it?

If the manufacturers, promoters, and trade associations want to defend the presence of toxins like fluoride, Monosodium Glutamate, Aspartame, and E. Coli in our food and drink, they can do so after these poisons have been removed.

Meanwhile, we will enjoy a hiatus from the chemicals and toxic bacteria that have been making the population of America sicker every year.

Diabetes, ADHD, Autism, Stroke, Obesity, Arthritis, Alzheimer's, Heart Attack, Birth Defects, Chronic Fatigue Syndrome, Parkinson's, Huntington's, Juvenile Kidney Failure, Variant Creutzfeldt-Jakob disease.

These are just a few of the many disorders and diseases that may see a dramatic reduction once fluoride, MSG, Aspartame and contaminated beef are no longer a part of the American Diet.

Consider for a moment, that we have rid ourselves of these toxins, what could be done to undo the damage? Is there anything available that can improve our health now that the toxins poisoning the nation have been identified?

---

[152] Henkel, John. 'Irradiation, a safe measure for safer food.' **FDA Consumer Magazine**. May-June 1998.

MSG has no value as nutrient or a preservative.   Its absence from food will not cause difficulties, only solve them.

What, however, will happen with the multi billion-dollar diet industry?   What can replace Aspartame in all the items that a dieting and diabetic nation need?

Surprisingly enough, Mother Nature provides not only the answers, but also the cures.   Unlike the toxins they will replace, these cures will not make big profits for anyone.

Stevia, the Sweet Taste of Nature

When the GD Searle travesty has been rectified, and Aspartame has been removed from the food and beverages of our poisoned nations, what will the dieters and diabetics do? They could do what the native people of Paraguay have done for 1500 years. They could turn to the leaves of the Stevia Rebaudiana plant. This plant grows wild and plentiful in South America. Its leaves have been found to be 30 times sweeter than sugar. When Stevia leaves are processed, they produce Stevia powder, (Stevioside) 300 times sweeter than sugar. The miracle is that Stevia sweetens without adding any calories, and it does so without harmful side effects.

Stevia goes even farther than just sweetening. Stevia has been thoroughly researched and found to help the body fight off gastrointestinal viruses and food borne bacteria, lower blood pressure in subjects with hypertension, and assist in insulin production in people with Type II diabetes. All this and a fine sweetener, too!

Tea made from Stevia leaves seems to have a protective effect inside the gastrointestinal system. Scientists have found that Stevia protects the gastric system from Rotoviruses, a common cause of diarrhea.[153]   This tea has also been found to destroy harmful

---

[153] Takahashi, K. Matsuda, M. Ohashi, K. Taniguchi, K. Nakagomi, O. Abe, Y. Mori, S. Sato, N. Okutani, K. Shigeta, S. "Analysis of anti-rotavirus activity of extract from Stevia rebaudiana." **Antiviral Res** 2001 Jan;49(1):15-24.

contagions in consumed food, specifically E-coli, the bacteria responsible for the poisoning of thousands of people in Walkerton, Ontario.

Those with hypertension could find assistance from Stevia. In a published research paper, 60 subjects with high blood pressure were given Stevia tablets 3 times daily for 3 months. The treatment significantly reduced their blood pressure and kept it lower 9 months after the experiment had ended. The study concluded its findings by saying that Stevia should be considered as an alternative therapy for patients with hypertension.[154]

For those with type II diabetes Stevia may bring hope. Researchers have shown that Stevia can stimulate pancreatic insulin production in Type II diabetic subjects.[155]

Unlike Aspartame, Stevia is a safe food sweetener. This fact has been well documented in hundreds of studies throughout the world. Research has shown that Stevia in large doses does not cause damage to DNA,[156] does not harmfully affect sexual reproductivity,[157] and is not carcinogenic.[158]

Millions of people in Japan have enjoyed the benefits of Stevia as a sweetener for the last 25 years. Currently China, Brazil, and South Korea have also approved widespread use of Stevia in products.

---

[154] Chan, P. Tomlinson, B. Chen, YJ. Liu, JC. Hsieh, MH. Cheng, JT. "A double-blind placebo-controlled study of the effectiveness and tolerability of oral stevioside in human hypertension." **Br J Clin Pharmacol** 2000 Sep;50(3):215-20.

[155] Jeppesen, PB. Gregersen, S. Poulsen, CR. Hermansen, K. "Stevioside acts directly on pancreatic beta cells to secrete insulin: actions independent of cyclic adenosine monophosphate and adenosine triphosphate-sensitive K+-channel activity." **Metabolism** 2000 Feb;49(2):208-14.

[156] Sekihashi, K. Saitoh, H. Sasaki, Y. "Genotoxicity studies of stevia extract and steviol by the comet assay." **J Toxicol Sci** 2002 Dec;27 Suppl 1:1-8.

[157] Aritajat, S. Kaweewat, K. Manosroi, J. Manosroi, A. "Dominant lethal test in rats treated with some plant extracts." **Southeast Asian J Trop Med Public Health** 2000;31 Suppl 1:171-3.

[158] Das, S. Das, AK. Murphy, RA. Punwani, IC. Nasution, MP. Kinghorn, AD. "Evaluation of the cariogenic potential of the intense natural sweeteners stevioside and rebaudioside." **Caries Res** 1992;26(5):363-6.

Unfortunately in the U.S. the FDA has declared it illegal to put Stevia in food. Like puppets, Canada's CFIA followed suit.

Why is it that a natural, beneficial substance is banned from America's food production?

Once again the answer is money. A single company cannot patent Stevia, being that it is a natural substance. Unlike Aspartame, whose profits benefit a single company, any manufacturer can produce and supply Stevia.

Rob McCaleb is the founder and President of the non- profit Herb Research Foundation, in Colorado. He has done a large amount of research and has a great deal to say about the use of Stevia. McCaleb discovered that the FDA ban on Stevia could be at the request of the company behind Nutrasweet. Now he complains that the FDA has made it harder for Stevia to be approved as a food additive than it was for Aspartame, which as we know from a previous chapter, violated numerous testing protocols and was approved under suspicious circumstances.

McCaleb points out the complete incompetence of the FDA, who deny Stevia's use in foods in America while American corporations like Coca Cola and Beatrice foods add it to the products they market in Japan and other countries.[159]

While other countries enjoy the benefits of Stevia, we suffer the side affects of Aspartame. The FDA has received more complaints about adverse reactions to Aspartame and MSG than almost any other chemical food additive on the American market.

Stevia has ended up on the government blacklist written by corporations bent on promoting profit over human health. Known toxins like fluoride, Aspartame and Monosodium Glutamate get full support while their victim's voices go unheard.

---

[159] McCaleb, Rob, http://www.holisticmed.com/sweet/stv-faq.txt, Herb Research Foundation.

The FDA, instead of being a force to protect the people from toxic substances, may have become the protector of corporate America's right to poison us and profit by it.

Melatonin, Nature's Healer for the Nation

Melatonin is a hormone found within the body. Its greatest influence is over the body's sleep cycle. It has however, another surprising ability. Melatonin is a powerful anti-oxidant. An anti-oxidant is a substance that binds to 'free radicals' in the human body. Free radicals are toxins that roam the body. They are highly reactive molecular chains that seek out other molecules to bind with. This binding can result in a harmful or even carcinogenic substance that can play havoc with the body's systems.

Anti-oxidants are like the body's police force, patrolling the blood, cells, tissues and organs of the brain. When they happen upon a free radical, they bond with it, tying its molecular arms so that it cannot cause any damage by binding with other locations.

Toxic chemicals like fluoride, along with unbound protein strands like Glutamate and aspartate, are free radicals. They are highly reactive substances that in large numbers can bind to chemicals, cells, and even neurons in the body to produce devastating effects. By injecting Monosodium Glutamate directly into the brain of a creature, scientists can cause massive destruction of the brain cells that this free radical comes in contact with. But when large amounts of Melatonin are present in the region that the MSG targets, the MSG fails to destroy the brain cells. Researchers have described the ability of Melatonin to stop the damage that MSG causes as a neuroprotective effect.[160]

The protective effects of Melatonin do not end with the brain. Since its discovery as a free radical scavenger in 1993, over 800 publications have confirmed Melatonin's ability to neutralize harmful molecules in the body.[161]

The pineal gland produces Melatonin naturally within the body. The chief role of Melatonin seems to be the creation of the natural sleep cycle of people and animals. During the day, people's Melatonin levels drop considerably, while in the evening this hormone becomes more prevalent in the blood. Melatonin counteracts dopamine, which is the hormone most utilized during the daytime hours. People with good sleep cycles show a balance between these two chemicals. However, the pineal gland loses its ability to create Melatonin as the body ages. This reduction in Melatonin levels can be linked to all manner of physical ailments. Luckily, synthetic Melatonin is easily available, and in studies has shown remarkable properties that improve all manner of physical conditions from insomnia to cancer.

---

[160] Espinar, A. Garcia-Oliva, A. Isorna, EM. Quesada, A. Prada, FA. Guerrero, JM. "Neuroprotection by melatonin from Glutamate-induced excitotoxicity during development of the cerebellum in the chick embryo." **J Pineal Res** 2000 Mar;28(2):81-8.

[161] Tan, DX. Reiter, RJ. Manchester, LC. Yan, MT. El-Sawi, M. Sainz, RM. Mayo, JC. Kohen, R. Allegra, M. Hardeland, R. "Chemical and physical properties and potential mechanisms: melatonin as a broad spectrum antioxidant and free radical scavenger." **Curr Top Med Chem** 2002 Feb;2(2):181-97.

Sleep Disorders

Since Melatonin is the natural hormone that induces sleep, ingesting a small dosage in tablet form is an effective cure for insomnia. Unlike prescription sleeping pills, it is not addictive, and allows a person to wake with no residual effects of drowsiness. Its use as a sleep aid has been documented in many areas of research. Melatonin has been used to help blind children establish a normal sleep pattern.[162] It has been used to successfully treat chronic insomnia in children.[163] It has even been used as an alternative to general anesthetic in children afraid to take an MRI.[164] Melatonin has been found to "be a safe, inexpensive, and a very effective treatment of sleep-wake cycle disorders," with no side effects or development of resistance to it.[165]

Pfizer, one of the worlds largest drug companies, offers Unisom SleepGels to help adults and children over 12 to fall asleep.

'www.rxlist.com' lists Unisom's side effects as:

> **General:** Urticaria, drug rash, anaphylactic shock, photosensitivity, excessive perspiration, chills, dryness of mouth, nose, and throat.

> **Cardiovascular System:** Hypotension, headache, palpitations, tachycardia, extrasystoles.

> **Hematologic System:** Hemolytic anemia, thrombocytopenia, agranulocytosis.

---

[162] Jan, JE. O'Donnell, ME. "Use of melatonin in the treatment of paediatric sleep disorders." J **Pineal Res** 1996 Nov;21(4):193-9.

[163] Smits, MG. Nagtegaal, EE. Van der Heijden, J. Coenen, AM. Kerkhof, GA. "Melatonin for chronic sleep onset insomnia in children: a randomized placebo-controlled trial." **J Child Neurol** 2001 Feb;16(2):86-92.

[164] Johnson, K. Page, A. Williams, H. Wassemer, E. Whitehouse, W. "The use of melatonin as an alternative to sedation in uncooperative children undergoing an MRI examination." **Clin Radiol** 2002 Jun;57(6):502-6.

[165] Jan JE, O'Donnell ME. "Use of melatonin in the treatment of pediatric sleep disorders." **J Pineal Res** 1996Nov;21(4):193-9.

Nervous System: Sedation, sleepiness, dizziness, disturbed coordination, fatigue, confusion, restlessness, excitation, nervousness, tremor, irritability, insomnia, euphoria, paresthesia, blurred vision, diplopia, vertigo, tinnitus, acute labyrinthitis, neuritis, convulsions.

GI System: Epigastric distress, anorexia, nausea, vomiting, diarrhea, constipation.

GU System: Urinary frequency, difficult urination, urinary retention, early menses.

Respiratory System: Thickening of bronchial secretions, tightness of chest and wheezing, nasal stuffiness.

Sometimes the side effects of a drug sound worse than the condition they are meant to prevent.

If Melatonin is such a successful sleep aid that is not addictive, has no side effects, and is gentle enough to use on children under of all ages, why aren't physicians prescribing it to the general public? Why instead do they prescribe drugs with long lists of side effects?

Money.

Have you ever been at a physician's office when a pharmaceutical sales person comes by? Have you seen all the free samples and little note pads that the doctors use? Those freebies come from drug companies. The drug companies are major funders of medical research. They even make large sums of money available to medical students to assist with their education.

What business do drug sales representatives have in a doctor's office?

They are there to sell their drug. They influence the choice of prescriptions that doctors make. How often have you gone into a doctor's office and come out with a suggestion instead of a prescription? Did the doctor ever tell you just to put some ice on it, a simple ointment, a bandage, or say that it will just get better on its own? Doctors give out prescriptions for many items that you can't get on the open shelf of a drug store. In many cases, the prescription is for a specific name of drug that only one company makes.

By practicing the prescription doctrine, physicians do their part to line the pockets of the pharmaceutical companies that help fund their profession.

The main reason that pharmaceutical companies fund research is to find a pill that can treat an ailment and that that pill can be patented to guarantee their exclusive right to profit from the drug.

The reason that physicians do not prescribe Melatonin to their sleep deprived patients is this:

No pharmaceutical company can make exclusive profit from it.

Melatonin is a naturally occurring hormone that cannot be patented by any company. It is inexpensive to produce. A four-month supply may cost you about ten dollars. At that price, how can a pharmaceutical company generate the kind of profit they are used to?

Sleep disorders are not the only thing that you won't see Melatonin prescribed for. Medical research has discovered over a dozen other ailments that can be treated by an inexpensive dose of Melatonin. From ulcers to bladder problems, epilepsy to cancer, reports published in scientific journals sing the praises of Melatonin, while the physicians across the country are silent.

Instead of healthy natural cures we are inundated with high priced drugs that have side effect lists that read like an encyclopedia.

The following sections outline the scientifically proven facts about Melatonin. These are the ailments that a simple, inexpensive cure may rectify. For those of you who are ready to take a stand against the profiteering of drug companies that bloat themselves at the price of our health, take this knowledge to your doctor and ask what single prescription medication can offer all these benefits without side effects and a thousand dollar-a-day price tag.

Gastrointestinal Disorders

Melatonin is a hormone that is essential to gastrointestinal health. It is found in this system at 10 to 100 times the concentration found in the blood. It has an important protective effect, and has been suggested in the treatment and prevention of gastric ulcers,[166] as well as "colorectal cancer, ulcerative colitis, gastric ulcers, irritable bowel syndrome, and childhood colic."[167] Perhaps there is a link between the increase in Crohn's and Colitis disease and the prevalence of MSG in the diet. Melatonin may be one form of treatment that could help those afflicted with these disorders.

More research in this direction is definitely needed.

Infant Toxicity

Septic shock is a very serious condition that some infants are born with. The baby is born with such a large amount of toxic elements in its system that little hope is offered to the parents. Many newborns with this condition die within a few days of delivery. Doctors at the University of Texas Health Science Center, San Antonio, gave ten septic babies large doses of Melatonin within 12 hours of birth. These babies had a survival rate of 100%, while the septic babies that did not receive Melatonin suffered a 30% mortality rate before they were four days old.[168]

Our hearts go out to the parents of these infants. Hopefully, this groundbreaking research will protect many more newborns to come.

---

[166] Singh, P. Bhargava, VK. Garg, SK. "Effect of melatonin and beta-carotene on indomethacin induced gastric mucosal injury." **Indian J Physiol Pharmacol** 2002 Apr;46(2):229-34.

[167] Bubenik GA. "Gastrointestinal melatonin: localization, function, and clinical relevance." **Dig Dis Sci** 2002 Oct;47(10):2336-48.

[168] Cardinali, DP. Ladizesky, MG. Boggio, V. Cutrera, RA. Mautalen, C. "Melatonin effects on bone: experimental facts and clinical perspectives." **J Pineal Res** 2003 Mar;34(2):81-7.

Attention Deficit Hyperactive Disorder

At seven years old, little Johnny was found to be more hyper than the other children. His mother could not get him to keep still. A veritable ball of energy, he was always bouncing from here to there, never able to keep focused on a task. The year was 1974, long before the invention of Ritalin. ADHD was not even a recognized condition then. Little Johnny's hyperactivity was not even formally diagnosed. His mother was desperate, and the doctor was only too willing to prescribe Phenobarbital, a serious anti-psychotic and highly addictive substance, to counteract his erratic behavior.

If only Johnny's mother had known what research shows now.

MSG intake during pregnancy may well have caused the condition that little Johnny suffered from. MSG in the adolescent diet could further aggravate the child's hyperactivity. ADHD is linked to a problem in the dopamine levels within the body.[169] Increased dopamine levels in the body are linked to the hyper active behaviors that ADHD children suffer. Currently Ritalin is the most commonly prescribed medication for reducing the actions of dopamine, but there is a better alternative. Dopamine can be naturally controlled by the introduction of increased Melatonin.[170]

By removing MSG and all food ingredients that contain Glutamate from the diet, and giving Melatonin time-release capsules to these ADHD children, a natural balance could occur between the two hormones, creating an equalibrium in the child. This could reduce both the level of hyperactivity and the difficulty with attention span that these children have.

How do I know that Melatonin and reduction in dietary Glutamate could cure ADHD?

---

[169] Arnold, LE. Pinkham, SM. Votolato, N. "Does zinc moderate essential fatty acid and amphetamine treatment of attention-deficit/hyperactivity disorder?" **J Child Adolesc Psychopharmacol** 2000 SUMMMER;10(2):111-7.

[170] Zisapel, N. "Melatonin-dopamine interactions: from basic neurochemistry to a clinical setting." **Cell Mol Neurobiol** 2001 Dec;21(6):605-16.

I was little Johnny. For thirty-five years my family has suffered from my hyperactive state.

A year ago I started taking Melatonin on a daily basis. By removing all sources of free-Glutamate from my diet, and leveling out my dopamine levels with melatonin, I have been able to completely reduce all symptoms of ADHD that I had. I now know the pleasure of sitting still, and the bliss of uninterrupted concentration.

We have two sons that are also ADHD possibly because of MSG. By giving them Melatonin and reducing their glutamate intake we are protecting them not only from further poisoning, but also from the following side effects of the Ritalin that doctors have been pushing on ADHD children:

- *drug addiction*
- *nervousness and insomnia*
- *nausea and vomiting*
- *dizziness*
- *headaches*
- *changes in heart rate and blood pressure (usually elevation of both, but occasionally depression)*
- *skin rashes and itching*
- *abdominal pain*
- *weight loss*
- *digestive problems*
- *toxic psychosis*
- *psychotic episodes*
- *severe depression upon withdrawal*
- *loss of appetite (may cause serious malnutrition)*
- *tremors and muscle twitching*
- *fevers, convulsions, and headaches (may be severe)*

- *irregular heartbeat and respiration (may be profound and life threatening)*

- *anxiety, restlessness*

- *paranoia, hallucinations, and delusions*

- *excessive repetition of movements and meaningless tasks*

- *while death due to non-medical use of Ritalin is not common, it has been known to occur.*

Narconon: www.drug-sideeffects.com/ritalin.htm

Very little is known about the way Ritalin (known as methylphenidate) affects ADHD symptoms. *"There is neither specific evidence which clearly establishes the mechanism whereby methylphenidate produces its mental and behavioral effects in children, nor conclusive evidence regarding how these effects relate to the condition of the central nervous system."*[171]

Not very reassuring words for a drug that doctors are passing out to children in record numbers.

The number of children diagnosed with this disorder grows each year, and every year the number of Ritalin prescriptions increase. While the bank accounts of the pharmaceutical giant Novartis (Ritalin's creator) are expanding, the pocket books of parents dealing with the disorder are shrinking. Ritalin prescriptions can be a life sentence. Children with ADHD carry it with them into adulthood.

The American Drug Enforcement Agency has targeted Ritalin as a drug that is widely abused.

> *"the primary legitimate medical use of methylphenidate (Ritalin®, Methylin®, Concerta®) is to treat attention deficit hyperactivity disorder (ADHD) in children. The increased use of this substance for the treatment of ADHD has paralleled an increase in its abuse among adolescents and young adults who crush these tablets and snort the powder to get high. Youngsters have little difficulty obtaining methylphenidate from classmates*

---

[171] RXLIST, Clinical Pharmacology. http://www.rxlist.com/cgi/generic/methphen_cp.htm.

or friends who have been prescribed it. Greater efforts to safeguard this medication at home and school are needed."

http://www.dea.gov/concern/methylphenidate.html

Ritalin could make the lives of ADHD children more difficult than they already are.

Melatonin, on the other hand, has documentation supporting its natural suppression of dopamine.[172] Unlike Ritalin, Melatonin is not addictive, cannot be used to get high, costs pennies to use, is found naturally in the body, and has none of the dangerous side effects that Ritalin has.

Melatonin has helped my two sons and myself to overcome the ADD and ADHD that has affected us. Melatonin supplements, along with the removal of glutamates from our diet, have created a dramatic change for the better.

It is a shame that physicians have not directed parents to a more natural and affordable way of treating ADHD. One that not only may prove more effective then Ritalin, but with far less side effects for the child as well.

Autism

Previous paragraphs in this book outlined the similarities between ADHD and autism. Research now suggests that the Melatonin that could help ADHD sufferers may also help those with autism as well. Individuals with autism have considerably lower levels of Melatonin in their bodies than healthy subjects.[173] This may cause many imbalances within the body's systems. Perhaps Melatonin

---

[172] Appenrodt, E. Schwarzberg, H. 'Methylphenidate-induced motor activity in rats: modulation by melatonin and vasopressin.' **Pharmacol Biochem Behav** 2003 Apr;75(1):67-73.

[173] Kulman, G. Lissoni, P. Rovelli, F. Roselli, MG. Brivio, F. Sequeri, P. "Evidence of pineal endocrine hypofunction in autistic children." **Neuroendocrinol Lett** 2000;21(1):31-34.

could be used to counteract some of the behaviors that are currently controlled by dangerous anti-psychotic drugs.

Currently there are no drugs specific to the treatment of autism. As a case manager for autistic individuals, I have sat in on many psychiatric appointments where the psychiatrists had no idea what medications to prescribe. With my 14 years experience working with people with autism, I have found these health-professionals often ask my opinion on what medication to prescribe. If only I had known about Melatonin.

Autistic individuals have been shown to have decreased Glutamate transport neurons in the brain.[174] They also have abnormally high amounts of Glutamate in the blood.[175] Research shows that there is a direct link between abnormal Glutamate receptors in the brain and the occurrence of autism.[176]

Since Melatonin has been shown to be a natural counter-agent to excess Glutamate, it would make Melatonin a logical treatment for Autism.

Individuals with autism have also shown a predisposition to sleep-disorders, and could benefit from the sleep inducing effects of Melatonin treatment.

Research into the use of Melatonin on people with autism may one day unlock a way to reverse the disorders debilitating effects.

---

[174] Purcell, AE. Jeon, OH. Zimmerman, AW. Blue, ME. Pevsner, J. "Postmortem brain abnormalities of the Glutamate neurotransmitter system in autism." **Neurology** 2001 Nov 13;57(9):1618-28.

[175] Fatemi, SH. Halt, AR. Stary, JM. Kanodia, R. Schulz, SC. Realmuto, GR. "Glutamic acid decarboxylase 65 and 67 kDa proteins are reduced in autistic parietal and cerebellar cortices." **Biol Psychiatry** 2002 Oct 15;52(8):805-10.

[176] Jamain, S. Betancur, C. Quach, H. Philippe, A. Fellous, M. Giros, B. Gillberg, C. Leboyer, M. Bourgeron, T. "Linkage and association of the Glutamate receptor 6 gene with autism." **Mol Psychiatry** 2002;7(3):302-10.

Stroke and Traumatic Brain Injury

Stacey was a bright young girl. She had worked hard in high school and graduated with excellent marks. She wanted to be a teacher and had been accepted into an excellent college for the fall semester. She never made it there. Stacey was a passenger in a horrendous car accident. Her friend behind the wheel died at the scene. She received a massive blow to her head.

At the hospital the surgeons worked quickly and with considerable expertise. It was too late. Blood vessels had broken within her brain, flooding vital areas with chemicals that the sensitive cells within the skull could not cope with.

When I first met Stacey she was at a sheltered workshop for the mentally handicapped, putting bolts into plastic bags. Instead of teaching she was now assisted by trainers, who had to remind her daily which table she sat at and which locker was hers. Though I saw her almost every day she always greeted me like I was a stranger she had never seen before. Her dreams of success were shattered by an injury that would shadow her and her family the rest of her life.

We are all only one accident away from that future.

Our minds are our most valuable commodity. The human body is designed to protect us from elements that could cause damage like the kind Stacey experienced. The blood brain barrier exists to protect the delicate inner workings of the brain from chemicals in the blood that could damage this system.

When Monosodium Glutamate in the blood enters the brain in unregulated amounts neurotoxicity occurs. Neural cells become over-excited by Glutamate or other excitotoxins and stimulate themselves to death. Research shows that both hemorrhagic stroke and accidental brain injury can allow this kind of brain damage to occur.

In the case of ischemic stroke, the blood supply to an area of the brain is cut off. Oxygen that regulates crucial chemical levels around the brain cells is in short supply. Harmful chemicals like nitric oxide and Glutamate can increase to dangerous levels. These chemicals are considered free radicals, and bond to nerve receptors and other molecules in the brain to cause irreparable damage.

In cases of traumatic brain injury, ischemic and hemorrhagic stroke, Melatonin can be highly effective at reducing the damage caused.[177]

The anti-oxidizing properties of Melatonin directly reduce the ability of free radicals to collect and harm the vulnerable structures in the brain. Melatonin injections given within two hours of a stroke dramatically decrease the permanent brain damage that the stroke would have caused.[178]

Melatonin is an effective protective agent, guarding the brain from damage caused by toxic levels of Glutamate in the brain. In a recent study it was discovered that Melatonin injected into the cerebellum of subjects created a protective effect against Glutamate injected into the same area, while Glutamate injected into the brain of untreated subjects caused neural cell death.[179]

Melatonin, used in the pretreatment of stroke victims, has been shown to reduce the severity of damage in successive strokes by as much as 46%. Motor, sensory memory, and psychological problems due to stroke could be reduced by treatment with Melatonin.[180]

Since Melatonin has been shown to be beneficial in reducing the severity of brain damage in both stroke and traumatic brain accident victims, perhaps it will become an early response

[177] Cheung, RT. "The utility of melatonin in reducing cerebral damage resulting from ischemia and reperfusion." **J Pineal Res** 2003 Apr;34(3):153-60.

[178] Pei, Z. Pang, SF. Cheung, RT. "Administration of melatonin after onset of ischemia reduces the volume of cerebral infarction in a rat middle cerebral artery occlusion stroke model." **Stroke** 2003 Mar;34(3):770-5.

[179] Espinar, A. Garcia-Oliva, A. Isorna, EM. Quesada, A. Prada, FA. Guerrero, JM. "Neuroprotection by melatonin from Glutamate-induced excitotoxity during development of the cerebellum in the chick embryo." **J Pineal Res** 2000 Mar;28(2):81-8.

[180] Kondoh, T. Uneyama, H. Nishino, H. Torii, K. "Melatonin reduces cerebral edema formation caused by transient forebrain ischemia in rats." **Life Sci** 2002 Dec 20;72(4-5):583-90.

treatment method used by emergency workers and first response teams everywhere. Melatonin has been proven to reduce the amount of permanent debilitating damage from a stroke or brain accident, wouldn't you be asking for it?

Research in this direction raises another question: if toxic levels of Glutamate entering the brain from broken blood vessels can cause increased brain damage in stroke and accident victims, would reducing the amount of Glutamate in your blood also reduce the level of damage that the victim suffers? Could current stroke or brain accident victims suffer less paralysis and brain damage if they had avoided MSG-laden food in the meal eaten just before their affliction struck them? More studies answering this question are definitely needed. I don't know about you, but until there is hard evidence to disprove my concern, I'm not taking any chances.

I see Stacey now and then, and she still doesn't remember who I am.

Epilepsy

Melatonin has been proven to defend the brain against attacks by excitotoxic chemicals.[181] MSG can cause epileptic convulsions. Because Melatonin directly counteracts the free radicals that could be the cause of the brain misfiring to induce epilepsy, it is possible that Melatonin could replace some of the current anti-convulsant medications on the market. Recent research has even gone as far as to compare the ability of Phenytoin (a commonly prescribed anti-convulsant drug sold under the brand name Dilantin) and Melatonin in reducing epileptic seizures. The findings of the

---

[181] Espinar, A. Garcia-Oliva, A. Isorna, EM. Quesada, A. Prada, FA. Guerrero, JM. "Neuroprotection by melatonin from Glutamate-induced excitotoxicity during development of the cerebellum in the chick embryo." **J Pineal Res** 2000 Mar;28(2):81-8.

research "showed a superior protective effect of Melatonin over Phenytoin."[182]

So why wouldn't Melatonin be prescribed for epilepsy instead of Dilantin?

Is Melatonin more dangerous to take than Phenytoin (Dilantin)? According to www.Rxlist.com, a website that lists drugs and their side effects and is sponsored by major pharmaceutical companies, Melatonin has the side effects of drowsiness, headache, or upset stomach. Rxlist reports that Dilantin has the following side effects:

> Nystagmus, ataxia, slurred speech, decreased coordination and mental confusion. Dizziness, insomnia, transient nervousness, motor twitchings and headache have also been observed as well as nausea, tardive dyskenesia, constipation, toxic hepatitis and liver damage. Skin rashes of various sorts including the possibly fatal forms of bullous, exfoliative or purpuric dermatitis, lupus erythematosus, Stevens-Johnson syndrome and toxic epidermal necrolysis. Also included is thrombocytopenia, leukopenia, granulocytopenia, agranulocytosis and pancytopenia with or without bone marrow suppression, Macrocytosis and megaloblastic anemia, Lymphadenopathy including benign lymph node hyperplasia, pseudolymphoma, lymphoma. Hodgkin's disease has also been reported. Add to these the side effects of coarsening of the facial features, enlargement of the lips, gingival hyperplasia, hypertrichosis and Peyronie's disease. Hypersensitivity syndrome (which may include, but is not limited to, symptoms such as arthralgias, eosinophilia, fever, liver dysfunction, lymphadenopathy or rash), systemic lupus erythematosus and immunoglobulin abnormalities.

'www.rxlist.com' goes on to report that pregnant women are at risk of having infants with a higher incidence of birth defects, including prenatal growth deficiency, microcephaly and mental deficiency.

---

[182] Srivastava, AK. Gupta, SK. Jain, S. Gupta, YK. "Effect of melatonin and phenytoin on an intracortical ferric chloride model of posttraumatic seizures in rats." **Methods Find Exp Clin Pharmacol** 2002 Apr;24(3):145-9.

Rxlist reports that overdosing on Melatonin can cause headache, drowsiness and upset stomach. An overdose of 2 to 5 grams of Dilantin is fatal.

So why would Melatonin be overlooked at the doctor's office, while prescriptions for Dilantin, even with all its side effects, are plentiful?

Money, money, money.

Melatonin is not a patented substance. It is inexpensive and no pharmaceutical company can monopolize it. No Melatonin salesmen visit the physician's office. No drug company will fund research of it or sing its praises to the FDA or other medical communities. Why would the drug companies support a plentiful and inexpensive cure, when they can profit from a patent they own?

Medication Side Effects

Not only can Melatonin replace some anti-seizure and anti-psychotic medications, it can also help against the side effects of them as well.

Tardive Dyskinesia is a prevalent side effect of many anti-seizure medications. Its symptoms include hand trembling and involuntary facial tics. Melatonin has been shown to both prevent and reduce Tardive Dyskinesia in test subjects.[183] People given Melatonin showed a remarkable decrease in the involuntary movements caused by Tardive Dyskinesia.[184]

---

[183] Naidu, PS. Singh, A. Kaur, P. Sandhir, R. Kulkarni, SK. "Possible mechanism of action in melatonin attenuation of haloperidol-induced orofacial dyskinesia." **Pharmacol Biochem Behav** 2003 Feb;74(3):641-8.

[184] Shamir, E. Barak, Y. Shalman, I. Laudon, M. Zisapel, N. Tarrasch, R. Elizur, A. Weizman, R. "Melatonin treatment for tardive dyskinesia: a double-blind, placebo-controlled, crossover study." **Arch Gen Psychiatry** 2001 Nov;58(11):1049-52.

Melatonin can even prevent the serious side effects caused by anti-cancer medications and the radiation therapy provided to cancer patients.

Doxorubicin is a commonly used anti-cancer drug whose side effects include "toxic effects on the cardiovascular system."[185] By treating subjects with Melatonin, researches found that Melatonin protected the cardiac system from the harmful side effects of Doxorubicin.[186]

Research has also discovered that healthy cells of subjects given whole body irradiation therapy were protected by Melatonin administered before the radiation.[187]

Since Melatonin can provide protection from medication and treatment side effects, shouldn't physicians be offering this information to patients who could benefit from it?

Alzheimer's

ADHD and autism are not the only neurodegenerative diseases that Melatonin can be helpful in treating. Both Alzheimer's and Parkinson's have been shown to be caused by free radicals like MSG. Melatonin's anti-oxidizing properties combat these free radicals, and in doing so could protect against the development of Alzheimer's.[188]

---

[185] Xu, MF. Ho, S. Qian, ZM. Tang, PL. "Melatonin protects against cardiac toxicity of doxorubicin in rat." **J Pineal Res** 2001 Nov;31(4):301-7.

[186] Xu, MF. Ho, S. Qian, ZM. Tang, PL. "Melatonin protects against cardiac toxicity of doxorubicin in rat." **J Pineal Res** 2001 Nov;31(4):301-7.

[187] Koc, M. Buyukokuroglu, ME. Taysi, S. "The effect of melatonin on peripheral blood cells during total body irradiation in rats." **Biol Pharm Bull** 2002 May;25(5):656-7.

[188] Pappolla, MA. Simovich, MJ. Bryant-Thomas, T. Chyan, YJ. Poeggeler, B. Dubocovich, M. Bick, R. Perry, G. Cruz-Sanchez, F. Smith, MA. "The neuroprotective activities of melatonin against the Alzheimer beta-protein are not mediated by melatonin membrane receptors." **J Pineal Res** 2002 Apr;32(3):135-42.

Elderly people who have chronically low blood sugar are candidates for the development of Alzheimer's. Perhaps by using Melatonin as a preventative treatment for this population, the occurrence of this degenerative disease could be substantially reduced.

In those patients who already have Alzheimer's, removal of free Glutamates such as MSG from their diet, along with the addition of Melatonin, could reduce the debilitating effects of the disorder.

Both Parkinson's and Huntington's disease can be linked to excess Glutamate levels in the brain. Since Melatonin has been shown to negate the excitotoxic effects of Glutamate,[189] its use as a treatment for people suffering these diseases should be more thoroughly studied.

Schizophrenia

Schizophrenia has been linked to abnormal Glutamate processes in the brain. With the reduced capacity of the schizophrenic mind to handle increased Glutamate in the brain, the Glutamate itself could cause the symptoms seen in the delusional episodes representative of the disorder.

In excess forms, Glutamate acts as a free radical and an excitotoxin. Melatonin is one of the most effective neutralizers of free radicals in the body. Melatonin has neuro- protective effects against Monosodium Glutamate's excitotoxic effects in the brain.[190]

---

[189] Espinar, A. Garcia-Oliva, A. Isorna, EM. Quesada, A. Prada, FA. Guerrero, JM. "Neuroprotection by melatonin from Glutamate-induced excitotoxicity during development of the cerebellum in the chick embryo." **J Pineal Res** 2000 Mar;28(2):81-8.

[190] Espinar, A. Garcia-Oliva, A. Isorna, EM. Quesada, A. Prada, FA. Guerrero, JM. "Neuroprotection by melatonin from Glutamate-induced excitotoxicity during development of the cerebellum in the chick embryo." **J Pineal Res** 2000 Mar;28(2):81-8.

Melatonin could act to neutralize the excess Glutamate in patients with schizophrenia, possibly reducing the episodes that disable them.

Research that tests the effectiveness of Melatonin on people with schizophrenia could lead to a new way to reduce the debilitating effects of this disorder.

Cholesterol, High Blood Pressure and Heart Disease

High cholesterol levels and high blood pressure are both indicators of an increased chance of cardiac arrest. Billions of dollars worth of medications are purchased each year to reduce both cholesterol and the blood pressure of people suffering from these conditions.

Melatonin has the amazing ability to solve both these problems at a substantial monetary savings to the medical system and insurance companies. Melatonin can reduce blood cholesterol levels by as much as 38 percent. This amount is substantial considering a 10-15 percent cholesterol reduction can result in a 20 to 30 percent reduction in heart attack risk.[191]

Melatonin's beneficial effects don't stop there. 90 minutes after taking Melatonin, the blood pressure of people with hypertension returns to normal levels.[192]

Research has even shown that Melatonin can reduce the tissue damage done after cardiac arrest, and may even be able to reverse it.[193]

---

[191] Sewerynek, E. "Melatonin and the cardiovascular system." **Neuroendocrinol Lett** 2002 Apr;23 Suppl 1:79-83.

[192] Sewerynek, E. "Melatonin and the cardiovascular system." **Neuroendocrinol Lett** 2002 Apr;23 Suppl 1:79-83.

[193] Reiter, RJ. Tan, DX. "Melatonin: a novel protective agent against oxidative injury of the ischemic/reperfused heart." **Cardiovasc Res** 2003 Apr;58(1):10-9.

How many people suffering from high blood pressure, high cholesterol and even cardiac arrest could be helped if their physicians put down their prescription pads and suggested that their patients add Melatonin to their nightly vitamin intake?

Fluoride Poisoning

Fluoride poisoning by industrial toxic waste is increasing on a global scale.[194]

As the union of the workers at the EPA headquarters stated, fluoride causes bone degeneration, neurotoxic effects in the brain, cancer and organ damage. Many of these disorders have been shown to be reversed by the anti-oxidizing effect of Melatonin.

The ability of the body to protect bone from degeneration can be augmented by increasing Melatonin.[195] This effect could be helpful against fluoride's effect of reducing bone strength and causing bone cancers.

Melatonin has a protective effect against loss of bone mass.[196] It actually increases bone mass and density, promoting greater bone strength.[197] The ability of Melatonin to act as a scavenger of bone

---

[194] Krishnamachari, KA. "Skeletal fluorosis in humans: a review of recent progress in the understanding of the disease." **Prog Food Nutr Sci** 1986;10(3-4):279-314.

[195] Koyama, H. Nakade, O. Takada, Y. Kaku, T. Lau, KH. "Melatonin at pharmacologic doses increases bone mass by suppressing resorption through down-regulation of the RANKL-mediated osteoclast formation and activation." **J Bone Miner Res** 2002 Jul;17(7):1219-29.

[196] Ostrowska Z, Kos-Kudla B, Marek B, Swietochowska E, Gorski J. "Assessment of the relationship between circadian variations of salivary melatonin levels and type I collagen metabolism in ostmenopausal obese women." **Neuroendocrinol Lett** 2001 Apr;22(2):121-7.

[197] Koyama, H. Nakade, O. Takada, Y. Kaku, T. Lau, KH. "Melatonin at pharmacologic doses increases bone mass by suppressing resorption through down-regulation of the RANKL-mediated osteoclast formation and activation." **J Bone Miner Res** 2002 Jul;17(7):1219-29.

debilitating free radicals can also add to its bone protective properties.[198]

By drinking water that has had the fluoride removed, degenerative skeletal fluorosis can be reversed.[199]

We have already seen the ability of Melatonin to fight toxic levels of poisons in the blood of infants; perhaps it may assist against the fluoride collecting in us as well. Melatonin could also protect the brain against the fluoride that the EPA employees have stated reduces the IQ levels of children.

The visual evidence of Melatonin's effects are much more compelling proof of its ability to counteract fluoride poisoning. Scientific research has proven that fluorosis, (the early warning sign that your child has been poisoned by fluoride) is not as irreversible as dentists lead you to believe.[200]

Instead of the expensive cosmetic treatments that dentists suggest, fluorosis can be reversed by a diet rich in vitamins and anti-oxidants.[201] As studies in hundreds of publications have shown, Melatonin is one of the most effective anti-oxidants available.[202]

Providing you immediately remove all sources of fluoride in your child's diet, and catch the poisoning in its early stages, it is possible to reverse the effects of the fluoride poisoning. Jessi's teeth once mottled and deformed by fluoride, have shown a

---

[198] Cardinali, DP. Ladizesky, MG. Boggio, V. Cutrera, RA. Mautalen, C. "Melatonin effects on bone: experimental facts and clinical perspectives." **J Pineal Res** 2003 Mar;34(2):81-7.

[199] Song, XK. "Therapeutic effect of low-fluorine drinking water on fluorosis of bone" **Zhonghua Yi Xue Za Zhi** 1989 Sep;69(9):491-2, 34.

[200] Gupta, SK. Gupta, RC. Seth, AK. "Reversal of clinical and dental fluorosis." **Indian Pediatr** 1994 Apr;31(4):439-43.

[201] Susheela, AK. Bhatnagar, M. "40 Reversal of fluoride induced cell injury through elimination of fluoride and consumption of diet rich in essential nutrients and antioxidants." **Mol Cell Biochem** 2002 May-Jun;234-235(1-2):335-40.

[202] Lopez-Burillo, S. Tan, DX. Mayo, JC. Sainz, RM. Manchester, LC. Reiter, RJ. "Melatonin, xanthurenic acid, resveratrol, EGCG, vitamin C and alpha-lipoic acid differentially reduce oxidative DNA damage induced by Fenton reagents: a study of their individual and synergistic actions." **J Pineal Res** 2003 May;34(4):269-277.

remarkable improvement over the past year. By removing fluoride from our drinking water and adding Melatonin to our nightly routine, we have reversed the fluorosis that inspired this book.

Jessi's smile is prettier than ever.

It's not too late for your children.[203] Your swift actions can see to that.

[203] Gupta, SK. Gupta, RC. Seth, AK. Gupta, A. "Reversal of fluorosis in children." **Acta Paediatr Jpn** 1996 Oct;38(5):513-9.

Melatonin, the Body's Cancer Cure

When my father called me with the news that he had cancer, I was devastated. He controlled his emotions far better than I, proving himself the eternal optimist. His prostate cancer was in the beginning stages and he chose radiation therapy instead of surgery. I would get constant phone updates from him. One day he told me that the pills he was taking were worth $1000 dollars a day. Thank goodness the Canadian health care system was footing the bill. The radiation therapy was hard on him, some days leaving him feeling him more ill than the cancer itself did.

With luck and a lot of prayer he pulled through. If only I'd known then what I know now, I might have saved him a lot of pain and suffering.

Along with all of the documented beneficial powers of Melatonin you have read about so far, it has another unique feature:

It can stop the development and spread of cancer.

Scientists all over the world have come to realize that the circadian light and dark cycle seems to have an affect on the ability of the human body to prevent cancer. The human body creates more Melatonin in darkness, less when there is light. There has been a discovery that in arctic populations who spend months in total darkness, the incidence of cancer is considerably lower than in industrialized areas.[204] It has also been noted that people who are totally blind show 31% less incidence of cancer than sighted people.[205]

Conversely, it has been found that people who continually work the night shift have a higher incidence of cancer.[206]

Our mothers told us that a good night sleep is the body's way of repairing itself. Research has finally proven what our mothers have known for years. Melatonin is created at night by the pineal gland. Melatonin is crucial for the body's fight against cancer and other forms of physical break down. Scientists have found that people with tumor causing cancers have lower Melatonin levels than healthy subjects.[207] It may well be the Melatonin that is reducing the onset of cancer. Rats that have had their pineal glands removed show a dramatic increase in cancer cell development, while treating them with Melatonin reduced the cancer occurrence.[208]

While some studies point to Melatonin creating a decrease in all tumor causing cancers, many focus on two cancers that Melatonin is extremely effective at preventing and treating: prostate and breast cancer. In my research, the only cancer that Melatonin doesn't seem to be effective against is Leukemia. Scientific experimentation at the University of McGill in Montreal, Canada has found that the herbal supplement Echinacea Purpurea has a

[204] Erren, TC. Piekarski, C. "Does winter darkness in the Artic protect against cancer? The melatonin hypothesis revisited." **Med Hypotheses** 1999 Jul;53(1):1-5.

[205] Feychting, M. Osterlund, B. Ahlbom, A. "Reduced cancer incidence among the blind." **Epidemiology** 1998 Sep;9(5):490-4.

[206] Anisimov, VN. "The light-dark regimen and cancer development." **Neuroendocrinol Lett** 2002 Jul;23 Suppl 2:28-36.

[207] Bartsch, C. Bartsch, H. "Melatonin in cancer patients and in tumor-bearing animals." **Adv Exp Med Biol** 1999;467:247-64.

[208] Tamarkin, L. Cohen, M. Roselle, D. Reichert, C. Lippman, M. Chabner, B. "Melatonin inhibition and pinealectomy enhancement of 7,12-dimethylbenz(a)anthracene-induced mammary tumors in the rat." **Cancer Res** 1981 Nov;41(11 Pt 1):4432-6.

profound effect in helping the body to overcome Leukemia.[209] Echinacea is yet another substance ignored by the medical community possibly due to the fact that no drug company can profit from it.

Prostate Cancer

As men age their prostate glands becomes more likely to develop cancerous cells, which can become life threatening malignant tumors. Scientists have shown that the Melatonin levels in men drop considerably as they enter the later stages of life.[210] Men who developed prostate cancers show a below average production level of Melatonin. Research suggests that a reduction in Melatonin may be related to the development and growth of prostate cancer.[211]

To determine the prostate cancer threat in men, doctors test the prostate-specific antigen (PSA) levels in the blood. Elevated levels of the PSA are sometimes the individual's first warning that they may have a prostate condition. Melatonin has been found to reduce the PSA count in the blood of subjects with prostate tumors. Melatonin was also found to have anti-tumor properties.[212]

Not only does Melatonin seem to stop the proliferation of androgen-specific cancer cells and metastatic tumor growth in the Prostate, but it may also reverse the cancer itself.[213]

---

[209] Currier, NL. Miller, SC. "Echinacea purpurea and melatonin augment natural-killer cells in leukemic mice and prolong life span." **J Altern Complement Med** 2001 Jun;7(3):241-51.

[210] Schulman, C. Lunenfeld, B. "The ageing male." **World J Urol** 2002 May;20(1):4-10.

[211] Bartsch, C. Bartsch, H. Fluchter, SH. Attanasio, A. Gupta, D. "Evidence for modulation of melatonin secretion in men with benign and malignant tumors of the prostate: relationship with the pituitary hormones." **J Pineal Res** 1985;2(2):121-32.

[212] Xi, SC. Siu, SW. Fong, SW. Shiu, SY. "Inhibition of androgen-sensitive LNCaP prostate cancer growth in vivo by melatonin: association of antiproliferative action of the pineal hormone with mt1 receptor protein expression." **Prostate** 2001 Jan 1;46(1):52-61.

[213] Lissoni, P. Cazzaniga, M. Tancini, G. Scardino, E. Musci, R. Barni, S. Maffezzini, M. Meroni, T. Rocco, F. Conti, A. Maestroni, G. "Reversal of clinical resistance to LHRH analogue in metastatic prostate cancer by the pineal hormone melatonin: efficacy of LHRH analogue plus melatonin in patients progressing on LHRH analogue alone." **Eur Urol** 1997;31(2):178-81.

Every year, almost 200,000 new cases of prostate cancer are diagnosed in the United States and Canada. This form of cancer is common in North America and Western Europe, but rare in Africa, South America and Asia. This fact makes me consider that this may be yet another disease that may have a link to our westernized diet and lifestyle. Every year, hundreds of thousands of men undergo painful prostate surgery and radiation treatments. In the process they use billions of dollars worth of hospitalization and medication.

Simply adding Melatonin to your vitamin regimen could reduce the cancerous activity in your prostate, or, better yet, reduce your chance of ever getting cancer at all. That would, however, deny the drug companies and the medical establishment their right to profit from your pain.

Would that be so wrong?

Breast Cancer

Men aren't alone in benefiting from the anti-cancer effects of Melatonin. Women as well can reap its benefits. Blind women, show a marked decrease in breast cancer, while women who work shift work and sleep opposite to normal darkness cycles show an increased susceptibility to breast cancer.[214] Melatonin is the main hormone whose production is directly dependent on light/dark circadian rhythms.

This has led many scientists to come to the conclusion that Melatonin may be useful in breast cancer therapy.[215]

Over 200,000 women in United States and Canada are diagnosed with breast cancer each year. These women will have to choose

---

[214] Glickman, G. Levin, R. Brainard, GC. "Ocular input for human melatonin regulation: relevance to breast cancer." **Neuroendocrinol Lett** 2002 Jul;23 Suppl 2:17-22.

[215] Dillon, DC. Easley, SE. Asch, BB. Cheney, RT. Brydon, L. Jockers, R. Winston, JS. Brooks, JS. Hurd, T. Asch, HL. "Differential expression of high-affinity melatonin receptors (MT1) in normal and malignant human breast tissue." **Am J Clin Pathol** 2002 Sep;118(3):451-8.

between the surgically invasive lumpectomy, mastectomy, chemo, or radiation therapies. Unfortunately, for over 40,000 of these women the disease will prove fatal.

Research has found that Melatonin actually suppresses the growth of existing tumor cells in women.[216] Further research on breast cancer shows that tumors can be reduced in size and number with the addition of Melatonin to the diet.[217]

The American Cancer Society's Webpage at 'www.cancer.org' has hormone therapies listed under its heading of Suggestions for Breast Cancer Treatment. I read the article with interest hoping to see mention of the natural hormone, Melatonin. Instead of the Melatonin that studies have shown can treat breast cancer, the society lists the following artificially created and patented prescription drugs: Tamoxifen (sold as Nolvadex) and Raloxifene (an estrogen blocker sold as Evista).

Not only do these drugs have dangerous side effects, but they are an expensive treatment as well.

A visit to 'www.drugstore.com' gives us an idea of just how much the pharmaceutical companies are charging for the treatment sponsored by the American Cancer Society.

Nolvadex   suggested dosage: 20-40mg daily
                   30 day supply @ 40 mgs daily: $214.76
                   Daily dosage price: $7.16

Evista   suggested dosage: one 60 mg tablet daily
                   30 day supply @ 60 mgs daily: $70.99
                   Daily dosage price: $2.37

[216] Yuan, L. Collins, AR. Dai, J. Dubocovich, ML. Hill, SM. "MT(1) melatonin receptor overexpression enhances the growth suppressive effect of melatonin in human breast cancer cells." **Mol Cell Endocrinol** 2002 Jun 28;192(1-2):147-56.

[217] Anisimov, VN. Alimova, IN. Baturin, DA. Popovich, IG. Zabezhinski, MA. Manton, KG. Semenchenko, AV. Yashin, AI. "The effect of melatonin treatment regimen on mammary adenocarcinoma development in HER-2/neu transgenic mice." **Int J Cancer** 2003 Jan 20;103(3):300-5.

Taken long term, these drugs are far from inexpensive. But if they save a life from cancer, then any price is worth it right? But what if there is actually little evidence that these two drugs are actually effective at treating breast cancer?

In 2002, the American Society of Clinical Oncology gathered to review the evidence of Tamoxifen and Raloxifene in treating cancer. Their report found that data reviewed *"do not as yet suggest that tamoxifen provides an overall health benefit or increases survival."* They further went on to say, *"use of tamoxifen combined with hormone replacement therapy or use of raloxifene ... to lower the risk of developing breast cancer is not recommended outside of a clinical trial setting."*[218]

Not recommended outside of a clinical setting? Yet these are the prescriptions of choice given by doctors to breast Cancer patients all over North America. These are the drugs supported by the American Cancer Society.

If a group of expert cancer physicians does not fully validate and support the use of these drugs for breast cancer treatment, why are women being told to take them?

Money.

Those snake oil salesmen in the doctor's office are doing one terrific job. Doctors today are so overworked by their caseloads, how can anyone expect them to keep up on the last pharmaceutical discoveries and published research. Instead they may listen to the recommendations of the American Cancer Society, who very well might receive funding directly from pharmaceutical companies. They may also rely on the research proposed to them in a 5-minute

[218] Chlebowski, RT. Col, N. Winer, EP. Collyar, DE. Cummings, SR. Vogel, VG. 3rd, Burstein, HJ. Eisen, A. Lipkus, I. Pfister, DG; American Society of Clinical Oncology Breast Cancer Technology Assessment Working Group. "American Society of Clinical Oncology technology assessment of pharmacologic interventions for breast cancer risk reduction including tamoxifen, raloxifene, and aromatase inhibition." **Clin Oncol** 2002 Aug 1;20(15):3328-43.

pitch from a professional looking salesman extolling the virtues of their soundly patented drug.

Can you trust a salesman to always tell the truth? Your health is not a used car.

Melatonin: Ignored in the U.S., Outlawed in Canada.

What company sales rep is out there visiting the physician's offices proclaiming the conclusive proof that Melatonin can benefit patients with cancer and the many other disorders that it may assist with? None. The lack of profit for an unpatented naturally available material causes it to be ignored by the medical community as a whole.

In the United States, though Melatonin can be found on the shelf of almost any drug store, doctors do not speak a word about its benefits. The labels on the bottles are required to state that Melatonin is a "product not intended to diagnose, treat, cure, or prevent disease."

There is more scientific evidence that Melatonin can treat, prevent, and even cure more ailments than almost any 'approved' prescription drug on the market.

If Melatonin sounds "too good to be true." It isn't. The truth is in the hundreds of independent studies made by doctors and medical researchers that do not profit from its promotion. The purpose of their research is to do what they were trained to do: help people.

Yet the benefits of Melatonin are ignored by governments and pharmaceutical companies alike.

In Canada Melatonin is considered a non-approved drug, and Canadians must buy it in the U.S. to be able to use it in Canada. Canada customs only allows them to import a three months supply at a time.

When I spoke to a representative at the Health Products and Food Branch about why Melatonin was not approved for use in Canada, he informed me that Melatonin, being a substance that has a natural purpose in the human body, was determined by the government to need further study before approval.

Further study? What about over 800 published articles that prove that Melatonin is a proven and beneficial protector against free-radical damage in the body?[219]

It looks like Canada's approval for a chemical has more to do with multi-national corporate influence than hard science. MSG, currently approved for unlimited addition to all foods in Canada, has over 1000 studies citing it as a toxin capable of causing obesity and brain cell death. Even Canada's own governmental research department admits that MSG stimulates many of the major organs of the body.[220]

Melatonin has not been found to be harmful to the human body.

In a shameful disregard for public safety, Canada has approved known toxins while barring Canadians from a natural substance that has been proven to benefit people suffering from stroke, sleep disorders, high blood pressure, epilepsy, side-effects from prescription drugs, and even cancer.

---

[219] Tan, DX. Reiter, RJ. Manchester, LC. Yan, MT. El-Sawi, M. Sainz, RM. Mayo, JC. Kohen, R. Allegra, M. Hardeland, R. "Chemical and physical properties and potential mechanisms: melatonin as a broad spectrum antioxidant and free radical scavenger." **Curr Top Med Chem** 2002Feb;2(2):181-97.

[220] Gill, SS. Mueller, RW. McGuire, PF. Pulido, OM. "Potential target sites in peripheral tissues for excitatory neurotransmission and excitotoxicity." **Toxicol Pathol** 2000 Mar-Apr;28(2):277-84. Bureau Chemical Safety, Health Protection Branch, Health Canada, Ottawa, Ontario.

Instead of offering us cures, Canada's government has legalized the toxic dumping of sodium fluoride in our water, promoted the addition of unlimited amounts of neurotoxic MSG into our food, offered us formaldehyde (in the form of Aspartame) in our diet foods, and allowed poisonous beef E. Coli into our food and water.

Melatonin and its myriad of health benefits are not available to a single patient in Canada. Canadian doctors have to turn a blind eye to the hundreds of published scientific studies showing Melatonin's benefits simply because the Canadian government decided that Melatonin poses more of a health risk than a known poison like sodium fluoride. While fluoride is a toxic prescription that the government has forced upon us, they will not even allow us the freedom to choose a proven cure.

To err is human, complete idiocy takes a government!

Pharmaceutical Companies: Profiting from the Unhealthy

The greatest profit from disease comes in the treatment, not the prevention or the cure.

If a drug company found a cure or a preventable cause of a disease, how much profit would they see?

Why sell one pill that can cure a disease, when you can sell a lifetime supply designed only to treat it. Forget about prevention. If a pharmaceutical company actually discovered that avoiding a toxin could eradicate the disease altogether (diabetes for instance), what money could they make from that?

It is not in the pharmaceutical company's best interest to make the public healthier. Their profit structure is designed to benefit from a more diseased one.

Pharmaceutical companies are now some of the largest and most profitable multinational companies in the world. They have become that way by being the largest drug pushers on the globe. Our asthmatic and ADHD children are hooked on their products from the earliest ages. Our elderly are pumped full of pills on a daily and nightly basis.

Industrial companies that fill our food and water supply with toxins are supporting the expansion and profiteering of the pharmaceutical companies.

More and more drug companies are involved in the creation of foods or substances that go directly into our food supply. Monsanto Corporation has both a drug division that supplies growth hormones to livestock, and a branch that designs genetically modified foods for human consumption. Pfizer and Novartis, two of the world's largest pharmaceutical companies, also make drugs that are given to the livestock used in America's food supply. Ajinomoto, the largest producer of MSG for use in food, is now venturing into the drug making industry.

Pharmaceutical company profits soar when the world's population grows increasingly unhealthy.

Considering that we are at our highest degree of medical knowledge, illnesses in the general population are at an all time high. How can this be? If the population of first century Europe was as sickly as ours is today, it is likely that the human race would have died out by the Middle Ages.

Will we make it to the next century?

Take Control

We do not live alone in this world. Surrounding us are the people we cherish, love, serve, and dedicate our lives to. Our parents made untold sacrifices so that we could live in a world free from hunger, war, disease and pain.

We desire to see our children protected from a world that is becoming more and more threatening. If only we could protect those we love from the harm that could befall them. If only we had the power to keep our loved ones from developing diseases like diabetes, Alzheimer's and cancer.

If we knew how to put an end to the threat these diseases had over us, we would do whatever possible to protect ourselves and those we love. Many of the things that endanger our health are all around us, a constant danger in our everyday lives.

Despite our technological advances, diseases and ailments that strike our population are at an all time high. Illnesses previously unheard of are now becoming epidemic in our nation.

The last century has brought vast changes, not only in industrial advancements, but also in the quality of air we breathe, water we drink and food we eat. Toxins and harmful substances never before seen in human history have begun to enter our bodies.

It is these poisons that currently threaten the health of our people, especially our children.

How is it that in America, with all its wealth and knowledge, we seem to have a more diseases and unfit population than that of the developing nations of the world?

We surround ourselves with the trappings of material success, thinking that we are giving our children the best of everything. Instead, we are giving them polluted air, toxic water and contaminated food.

For all our diligence as parents we have not been able to offer our children the safe world that we desire for them. Certainly if we were aware of the poisons that threaten our children, we would act quickly to remove the threat. We know about the dangers of lead, asbestos, arsenic, and mercury. What is it that we are missing? What unidentified toxic chemicals are making the current American population into diseased, infirm, and dependant on record numbers of prescription drugs?

It is not through lack of care or negligence that poisons are striking at our children and ourselves. It is due instead to something far more ominous than terrorism or the nuclear threat.

The reason that these toxins are slipping past our guard is because of careful promotion and manipulation of information. The poisons that could be the greatest threat to our health are actually being hailed as great industrial achievements: Sodium fluoride, Monosodium Glutamate and Aspartame.

Misinformation is not just the tool of communist regimes and dictators.

Corporate America has become the master of public influence, carefully marketing both their products and their pollutants as items that are beneficial to the population. The creators of these poisons are writing laws that protect their industry's profit margins, caring nothing for the people that laws were meant to protect.

The truth about these toxins poisoning millions in America is not shrouded in secrecy. It is not hidden away in vaults for no one to see. The truth about these poisons has already been brought to the attention of the governments that have the power to put a stop to them.

Arm yourself with the knowledge held in the pages of this book.

Make the changes in your lifestyle to prevent the onslaught of ailment and disease that these toxins cause.

Politicians and corporations may not hear your voice, but they will feel your choice.

Choose not to drink water adulterated with industrial waste.

Choose not to add to the profit of food manufacturers and pharmaceutical companies that promote the use of substances with toxic side effects.

Choose to read the ingredient list of processed foods and restaurant items. Make an informed choice of what goes into your mouth and the mouths of your children.

Refuse to be sheep fleeced by corporate America.

What you do now can save you and your children from being victims of the slow poisoning of America.

The Slow Poisoning of Mankind

A Report on the Toxic Effects of the Food Additive Monosodium Glutamate

Presented by John Erb to

Dr. Jorgen Schlundt, Director of Food Safety for the United Nations World Health Organization August 2006.

The Canadian Senate Committee on Autism, December 2006.

The Autism Interagency Committee of United States, November 2007.

Dr. Von Eschenbach, Commissioner of the Food and Drug Agency of the United States, December 2007.

Abstract:

Monosodium Glutamate was patented for use in food in 1909 by the Ajinomoto corporation of Japan. It saw limited use up until World War II when it was added to the rations of the Japanese troops. After the war it was introduced to America at the Chicago food Symposium of 1950. Restaurateurs such as Colonel Sanders and Food Manufacturers like Kraft, Campbell's and Heinz soon discovered that adding MSG to food was an inexpensive way to make it taste better, and it had the advantage of making people eat more.

Since 1950, the MSG use in the United States and countries with a westernized diet has grown dramatically. During the last six decades the occurrence of obesity, diabetes and Autism Spectrum Disorder have also increased.

This report gathers together published medical studies to determine what ailments MSG (Monosodium Glutamate) can be linked to. The evidence shows that Glutamate can be linked to a wide variety of ailments such as epilepsy, CNS and brain damage, eye cell damage, triggering obesity, diabetes, liver damage, adult-onset olivopontocerebellar degeneration, amyotrophic lateral sclerosis (ALS) and Autism.

In light of the overwhelming evidence showing the detrimental effects of the food additive Monosodium Glutamate it is requested that the Joint Food and Agriculture Committee/World Health Organization Expert Committee on Food Additives, the United States Food and Drug Agency, the United Kingdom Food Standards agency, and the European Food Safety Agency remove Monosodium Glutamate (and artificial ingredients that contain Glutamate) from the allowable additives list of their respective countries, and the Codex Alimentarius, and have Glutamate banned from vaccines as well.

Human Exposure

Orally:

Monosodium Glutamate is found in unlimited amounts in a wide variety of packaged foods. The list of foods it can be found in is listed in Appendix A. MSG is also added in unlimited amounts in restaurant and industrial food such as hospitals, retirement homes and cafeterias. Because food processors and manufacturers do not have to list the amount of MSG on their packaging, we have no way of knowing what a normal person or child would ingest in a days period. According to industry research 0.6% MSG added to food is optimal for making people eat progressively more and faster (Bellisle F, Monneuse MO, 1991). If this is the case, as much as .6% of a person's daily diet could be made up of MSG. In a daily intake of 2kgs of laced food the adult or child would receive a 12 gram dose of Monosodium Glutamate. A 12 gram dosage of MSG is lethal to a one kg rat. *JECFA Toxicology Study, FAO Nutrition Meetings Report Series,1974, No. 53*

Subcutaneously:

Though previous JECFA reports have disallowed MSG in foods for infants or those under one year of age, many infants and children receive doses of MSG in a variety of vaccinations. See Appendix C.

Air Transmission:

MSG is now being sprayed on crops and can become airborne. Though the Codex Alimentarius specifically disallows MSG's addition to fresh fruits and vegetables *(GFSA Annex to Table 3)* Auxigro, with 30% MSG content, has been approved by some countries to be sprayed on crops of fresh fruits and vegetables. Airborne effects of MSG sprays have not been studied by the JECFA.

Biological Aspects

Monosodium Glutamate is an amino acid readily utilized by glutamate receptors throughout the mammalian body. These glutamate receptors are present in the central nervous system as the major mediators of excitatory neurotransmission and excitotoxicity. Neural injury associated with trauma, stroke, epilepsy, and many neurodegenerative diseases such as Alzheimer's, Huntington's and Parkinson's diseases and amyotrophic lateral sclerosis may be mediated by excessive activation of the glutamate receptors. Neurotoxicity associated with excitatory amino acids encountered in food, such as monosodium glutamate, has also been linked to glutamate receptors. Glutamate receptors are found in the rat and monkey heart, the conducting system, nerve terminals and cardiac ganglia. They are also present in the kidney, liver, lung, spleen and testis. Therefore, food safety assessment should consider these tissues as potential target sites.

Potential target sites in peripheral tissues for excitatory neurotransmission and excitotoxicity.
Gill SS, Mueller RW, McGuire PF, Pulido OM.
Bureau of Chemical Safety, Health Protection Branch, Health Canada, Ottawa.
Toxicol Pathol. 2000 Mar-Apr;28(2):277-84

Short-term toxicity of Monosodium Glutamate

MSG Used to Trigger Epileptic Seizures

Epileptic convulsions were triggered in rats using small single doses of Monosodium Glutamate.

"Convulsive activity in 3, 10, 60 and 180-day old Sprague-Dawley rats was studied following the i.p. administration of 4 mg g-1 of commercial MSG. The latency period increased with the age of the animals while the duration of the convulsive period was longer in younger animals and shorter in 60-day old rats. Convulsions were predominantly tonic in 3 and 10-day old rats, tonic-clonic in 60-day old rats, and predominantly clonic in 180-day old animals. **The severity of the convulsions and death incidence increased progressively with age.**

Monosodium-L-glutamate-induced Convulsions--I. Differences in seizure pattern and duration of effect as a function of age in rats.
Arauz-Contreras J, Feria-Velasco A.
Gen Pharmacol. 1984;15(5):391-5.

"Adult rats (60 days old) were injected intraperitoneally with 5 mg/g monosodium L-glutamate (MSG). During the convulsive period (1 h after injection), uptake and release of [3H]norepinephrine (3H-NE) and [14C]dopamine (14C-DA) were measured. Data suggest that catecholaminergic **neurotransmission may play an important role in the etiopathology of convulsions in the experimental model using MSG.**"

Monosodium L-glutamate-induced convulsions: changes in uptake and release of catecholamines in cerebral cortex and caudate nucleus of adult rats.
Beas-Zarate C, Schliebs R, Morales-Villagran A, Feria-Velasco A.
Epilepsy Res. 1989 Jul-Aug;4(1):20-7.

MSG Used to Trigger CNS and Brain Damage

Single doses of MSG have been used to cause CNS and brain damage in rodents and chicks.

"Monosodium glutamate (MSG) was used to create a lesion in the CNS of the infant rat. Subcutaneous injections of MSG in four day old rat pups caused a high degree of cell necrosis in the arcuate nucleus of the hypothalamus"

Reaction of the hypothalamic ventricular lining following systemic administration of MSG.
Rascher K, Mestres P.
Scan Electron Microsc. 1980;(3):457-64.

"Administration of doses of glutamate (Glu) leads to selective neurodegeneration in discrete brain regions near circumventriclular organs of the early postnatal mouse. The arcuate nucleus-median eminence complex (ARC-ME) appears to be the most Glu-sensitive of these brain regions, perhaps because of the intimate relationships between its neurons and specialized astroglial tanycytes. A dose of 0.2 mg MSG/g BW s.c. causes clear but discrete injury to specific subependymal neurons of undetermined phenotype near the base of the third ventricle. Slightly higher doses of MSG evoke damage of additional neurons confined to the ventral region of the ARC traversed by tanycytes."

Exogenous glutamate enhances glutamate receptor subunit expression during selective neuronal injury in the ventral arcuate nucleus of postnatal mice.
Hu L, Fernstrom JD, Goldsmith PC.
Neuroendocrinology. 1998 Aug;68(2):77-88

"Various dosages of monosodium glutamate (M.S.G.) were injected to 5 day old male chicks. Body weights, food intake, rate of obesity, semen production, some endocrine criteria and brain pathology were studied til 235 days post injection. **All M.S.G. treated birds showed brain damage** in the rotundus nuclei, and in the area located dorsolaterally to the ventromedial hypothalamic nuclei (V.M.H.). In some of the M.S.G. treated birds, additional brain regions were damaged, i.e. V.M.H., mammillary nuclei, dorsomedial anterior nuclei, ovoid nuclei, subrotundus nuclei, archistriatum and lateral forebrain bundles."

The relation between monosodium
glutamate inducing brain damage, and
body weight, food intake, semen production
and endocrine criteria in the fowl.
Robinzon B, Snapir N, Perek M.
Poult Sci. 1975 Jan;54(1):234-41.

MSG Used to Damage Eye Cells in Vivo and in Vitro

Single doses of MSG have been used to trigger damage to various structures of the eye.

"**Monosodium L-glutamate is known to cause intracellular swelling, necrosis, and disappearance of most inner retinal neurons, with concomitant thinning of inner retinal layers within hours** after subcutaneous injection into neonatal rodents. A similar process can be observed in adult rat retina after intravitreal glutamate injection. To better describe and compare this process with that reported after systemic application, adult Sprague-Dawley rat eyes were intravitreally injected with 1 mumol monosodium L-glutamate and the retinas studied by LM and EM over a 2-month period. Results demonstrated that adult rat retina experienced severe degenerative changes which progressed in two stages: an initial stage of massive intracellular swelling and a second stage of necrosis and cell loss."

Histologic changes in the inner retina of
albino rats following intravitreal
injection of monosodium L-glutamate.
Sisk DR, Kuwabara T.
Graefes Arch Clin Exp Ophthalmol.
1985;223(5):250-8.

"**Monosodium glutamate added to 12-day chick embryo retinas in culture causes severe morphologic damage** to the retina as judged by light microscopic examination. Damage is evident after a few hours with concentrations as low as 0.3 mM. Glutamyltransferase induction is also appreciably inhibited by the amino acid. General protein synthesis and RNA synthesis appear to be less affected."

Effects of monosodium glutamate on chick
embryo retina in culture.
Reif-Lehrer L, Bergenthal J, Hanninen L.
Invest Ophthalmol. 1975 Feb;14(2):114-24.

Long-term toxicity of Monosodium Glutamate

MSG Used to Create Obese Test Subjects

In studies of new diet and diabetes drugs and treatments, a test subject must be used that will exhibit the characteristics of obesity and hyperinsulinemea. For scientists to create replicable results the factor that triggers obesity in the experimental test group must be 100% replicable. For guaranteed results researchers regularly use injections of MSG subcutaneously on test subjects on the day of birth or shortly thereafter

"Monosodium glutamate (MSG) was administered by various methods to mice and rats of various ages and the incidence of obesity was later measured. Newborn mice were injected subcutaneously with 3 mg MSG/g body-weight at 1, 2, 3, 6, 7, and 8 d of age; 16% died before weaning. Of the survivors, 90% or more became markedly obese. The proposed schedule of **injections in the newborn was almost 100% reliable in inducing a high extent of adiposity.** "

The induction of obesity in rodents by means of monosodium glutamate.
Bunyan J, Murrell EA, Shah PP.
Br J Nutr. 1976 Jan;35(1):25-39.

This replicable finding has been given the names 'monosodium glutamate obese rat' or 'MSG treated rat'.

Here are a few of the hundreds of studies that have used the rodent scientifically categorized as the MSG Treated Rat, a term synonymous with obesity, lethargy and hyperinsulinaemia:

Effect of adrenalectomy on the activity of small intestine enzymes in
monosodium glutamate obese rats.
Mozes S, Sefcikov Z, Lenhardt L, Racek L. Physiol Res. 2004;53(4):415-22.

Effect of fasting and refeeding on duodenal alkaline phosphatase activity in monosodium glutamate obese rats.
Racek L, Lenhardt L, Mozes S. Physiol Res. 2001;50(4):365-72.

Decreased lipolysis and enhanced glycerol and glucose utilization by adipose tissue prior to development of obesity in monosodium glutamate (MSG) treated-rats.
Dolnikoff M, Martin-Hidalgo A, Machado UF, Lima FB, Herrera E. Int J Obes Relat Metab Disord. 2001 Mar;25(3):426-33

Effects of chronic administration of sibutramine on body weight, food intake and motor activity in neonatally monosodium glutamate-treated obese female rats: relationship of antiobesity effect with monoamines.
Nakagawa T, Ukai K, Ohyama T, Gomita Y, Okamura H.
Exp Anim. 2000 Oct;49(4):239-49.

Effects of monosodium glutamate-induced obesity in spontaneously hypertensive rats vs. Wistar Kyoto rats: serum leptin and blood flow to brown adipose tissue.
Iwase M, Ichikawa K, Tashiro K, Iino K, Shinohara N, Ibayashi S, Yoshinari M, Fujishima M.
Hypertens Res. 2000 Sep;23(5):503-10.

Obesity induced by neonatal monosodium glutamate treatment in spontaneously hypertensive rats: an animal model of multiple risk factors.
Iwase M, Yamamoto M, Iino K, Ichikawa K, Shinohara N, Yoshinari M, Fujishima M.
Hypertens Res. 1998 Mar;21(1):1-6.

MSG Linked to Obesity in Humans

Research has shown a link between people who add MSG to their food and an increase in BMI.

"Animal studies indicate that monosodium glutamate (MSG) can induce hypothalamic lesions and leptin resistance, possibly influencing energy balance, leading to overweight. This study examines the association between MSG intake and overweight in humans. We conducted a cross-sectional study involving 752 healthy Chinese (48.7% women), aged 40-59 years, randomly sampled from three rural villages in north and south China. With adjustment for potential confounders including physical activity and total energy intake, MSG intake was positively related to BMI. Prevalence of overweight was significantly higher in MSG users than nonusers. **This research provides data that MSG intake may be associated with increased risk of overweight independent of physical activity and total energy intake in humans.**

Association of Monosodium Glutamate
Intake With Overweight in Chinese Adults:
The INTERMAP Study.
Ka He, Liancheng Zhao, Martha L Daviglus,
Alan R Dyer, Linda Van Horn, Daniel
Garside, Liguang Zhu, Dongshuang Guo,
Yangfeng Wu, Beifan Zhou, Jeremiah Stamler
Obesity (2008)

The Ways in Which MSG Triggers Obesity In Test Subjects:

MSG increases the appetite.

MSG added to food of sheep has resulted in an increase in appetite:

"Sheep with oesophageal fistulas were used in sham-feeding experiments to assess how sham intakes were affected by additions of monosodium glutamate (MSG) to the various straw diets. MSG at 5-40 g/kg fine and coarse ground straw increased sham intakes by 146% (P = 0.04) and 164% (P = 0.01) respectively. These findings indicated that **the intakes of poor-quality diets can be increased by improving their palatability with MSG.**"

Factors affecting the voluntary intake of
food by sheep. The effect of monosodium
glutamate on the palatability of straw diets
by sham-fed and normal animals.
Colucci PE, Grovum WL.
Br J Nutr. 1993 Jan;69(1):37-47.

MSG alters rat's ability to regulate food intake:

"Caloric regulation and the development of obesity were examined in rats which had received parenteral injections of monosodium glutamate (MSG) as neonates. Rats were injected with either 2 mg/g or 4 mg/g MSG on alternate days for the first 20 days of life. In adulthood, the ability to regulate caloric intake was tested by allowing animals access to diets of varying caloric densities. While control animals maintained relatively constant caloric intakes across dietary conditions, MSG-treated animals demonstrated an inability to respond to caloric challenges. **Treated animals decreased caloric intake on a diluted diet and consumed more calories** than controls when presented with a calorically dense diet."

Juvenile-onset obesity and deficits in caloric regulation in MSG-treated rats.
Kanarek RB, Meyers J, Meade RG, Mayer J.
Pharmacol Biochem Behav. 1979 May;10(5):717-21

A connection can be found in human test subjects: Two findings with MSG and human appetite are discovered:
1. When a human subject eats a meal with MSG, they become hungry again, sooner.
2. Humans will eat more food laced with MSG than control food without it.

"Subjects consumed soup preloads of a fixed size containing different concentrations of monosodium L-glutamate (MSG). Effects on appetite following these preloads, and when no soup was consumed, were assessed in 3 studies.The most important finding concerning MSG showed that motivation to eat recovered more rapidly following a lunchtime meal in which MSG-supplemented soup was served."

**Umami and appetite: effects of
monosodium glutamate on hunger and
food intake in human subjects.**
Rogers PJ, Blundell JE.
Physiol Behav. 1990 Dec;48(6):801-4.

"MSG's effects on the palatability of two experimental foods
were investigated in 36 healthy young men and women.
MSG improved palatability ratings, with an optimum at
0.6%. Weekly tests of free intake showed that subjects fed
the experimental foods with 0.6% MSG added ate
progressively more and faster, indicating increasing
palatability with repeated exposure. MSG facilitated intake
of some but not all target foods, and was associated with
positive (increased calcium and magnesium intake) or
adverse (increased fat intake) nutritional effects. It is
concluded that MSG can act as a palatability enhancer in the
context of the French diet. **It can facilitate long-term intake
in both young and elderly persons but it should be
utilized cautiously so as to improve nutrition**.

**Monosodium glutamate as a palatability
enhancer in the European diet.**
Bellisle F, Monneuse MO, Chabert M, Larue-
Achagiotis C, Lanteaume MT, Louis-
Sylvestre J.
Physiol Behav. 1991 May;49(5):869-73.

MSG increases the secretion of Insulin.

MSG has been shown in rats to over stimulate the pancreas
resulting in hyperinsulinemia. The excess insulin in the blood
increases the conversion of glucose into adipose tissue.

"Early postnatal administration of monosodium glutamate
(MSG) to rats induces obesity, hyperinsulinemia and
hyperglycemia in adulthood, thus suggesting the presence of

insulin resistance. We therefore investigated the effects of insulin on glucose transport and lipogenesis in adipocytes as well as insulin binding to specific receptors in the liver, skeletal muscle and fat tissues. **An increase of plasma insulin was found in 3-month-old rats treated with MSG during the postnatal period"**

Late effects of postnatal administration of monosodium glutamate on insulin action in adult rats.
Macho L, Fickova M, Jezova, Zorad S.
Physiol Res. 2000;49 Suppl 1:S79-85.

Even just adding MSG to the mouth of a rat can trigger an increase in insulin release:

"When the oral cavity was infused by MSG solution, a transient increase in blood insulin level was recognized at 3 min after this oral stimulation. These observations support the conclusion that taste stimulation of MSG induces cephalic-phase insulin secretion."

Cephalic-phase insulin release induced by taste stimulus of monosodium glutamate (umami taste).
Niijima A, Togiyama T, Adachi A.
Physiol Behav. 1990 Dec;48(6):905-8.

A connection can be found in human test subjects:

"To further study glutamate metabolism, we administered 150 mg/kg body wt of monosodium glutamate (MSG) and placebo to seven male subjects who then either rested or exercised. **MSG administration resulted in elevated insulin levels."**

**Glutamate ingestion and its effects at rest
and during exercise in humans.**
Mourtzakis M, Graham TE.
J Appl Physiol. 2002 Oct;93(4):1251-9.

"Monosodium (L)-glutamate (10 g) was given orally in a double-blind placebo-controlled cross-over study to 18 healthy volunteers, aged 19-28 years, with an oral (75 g) glucose load. CONCLUSIONS: **Oral (L)-glutamate enhances glucose-induced insulin secretion in healthy volunteers in a concentration-dependent manner.**"

**Effects of oral monosodium (L)-glutamate
on insulin secretion and
glucose tolerance in healthy volunteers.**
Chevassus H, Renard E, Bertrand G,
Mourand I, Puech R,Molinier N,
Bockaert J, Petit P, Bringer J.
Br J Clin Pharmacol. 2002 Jun;53(6):641-3.

MSG reduces the excretion of Ketones.

MSG has been shown in rats to reduce Ketone secretion, resulting in an obese rat with a propensity for creating adipose tissue(fat):

"MSG-treated rats showed shorter naso-anal and tail length, and a more marked intraperitoneal fat deposition than control rats. Plasma levels of **total ketone bodies were decreased in the MSG-treated rats as compared to control rats.**"

**Decreased ketonaemia in the monosodium
glutamate-induced obese rats.**
Nakai T, Tamai T, Takai H, Hayashi S,
Fujiwara R, Miyabo S.
Life Sci. 1986 Jun 2;38(22):2009-13.

A connection can be found in human test subjects:

"Production and use of ketone bodies are lower in obese women than in lean controls."

Ketone body metabolism in lean and obese women.
Vice E, Privette JD, Hickner RC, Barakat HA.
Metabolism. 2005 Nov;54(11):1542-5.

MSG reduces the excretion of Growth Hormone (GH) during adolescence.

MSG has been shown in rats to reduce Growth Hormone secretion, resulting in an obese rat with stunted stature:

Rats were treated with monosodium glutamate (MSG), 4 mg/g on alternate days for the first 10 days of life, to induce lesions of the arcuate nucleus and **destroy the majority of growth hormone-releasing hormone (GHRH) neurones**.

Depletion of hypothalamic growth hormone-releasing hormone by neonatal monosodium glutamate treatment reveals an inhibitory effect of betamethasone on growth hormone secretion in adult rats.
Corder R, Saudan P, Mazlan M, McLean C, Gaillard RC.
Neuroendocrinology. 1990 Jan;51(1):85-92.

A connection can be found in human test subjects:

In obese individuals, ...GH secretion is impaired without an organic pituitary disease and the severity of the secretory defect is proportional to the degree of obesity.

**Growth hormone status in morbidly obese
subjects and correlation with body
composition.**
Savastano S, Di Somma C, Belfiore A, Guida
B, Orio F Jr, Rota F,
Savanelli MC, Cascella T, Mentone A,
Angrisani L, Lombardi G, Colao A.
J Endocrinol Invest. 2006 Jun;29(6):536-43.

A recent study compared data from both humans and rats fed
MSG prenatally through the mother's diet, and made the
following recommendation:

> **"Oral administration of MSG to pregnant rats affects
> birth weight of the offspring**, and reduces GH serum levels
> are lowered in animals that received MSG during prenatal
> life via maternal feeding.....The flavouring agent MSG--at
> concentrations that only slightly surpass those found in
> everyday human food, exhibits significant potential for
> damaging the hypothalamic regulation of appetite, and
> thereby determines the propensity of world-wide obesity. **We
> suggest to reconsider the recommended daily allowances
> of amino acids and nutritional protein, and to abstain
> from the popular protein-rich diets, and particularly** from
> adding the flavouring agents MSG."

**Obesity, voracity, and short stature: the
impact of glutamate on the regulation of
appetite.**
Hermanussen M, Garcia AP, Sunder M, Voigt
M, Salazar V, Tresguerres JA.
Eur J Clin Nutr. 2006 Jan;60(1):25-31.

MSG Triggers Diabetes In Test Subjects:

The food additive Monosodium Glutamate is used to purposely create Diabetic rodents:

"The number of diabetic patients is increasing every year, and new model animals are required to study the diverse aspects of this disease. An experimental obese animal model has reportedly been obtained by injecting monosodium glutamate (MSG) to a mouse. We found that ICR-MSG mice on which the same method was used developed glycosuria. Both female and male mice were observed to be obese but had no polyphagia, and were glycosuric by 29 weeks of age, with males having an especially high rate of incidence (70.0%). Their blood concentrations of glucose, insulin, total cholesterol, and triglycerides were higher than in the control mice at 29 weeks. These high concentrations appeared in younger males more often than in females, and were severe in adult males. Also, the mice at 54 weeks of age showed obvious obesity and increased concentrations of glucose, insulin, and total cholesterol in the blood. The pathological study of ICR-MSG female and male mice at 29 weeks of age showed hypertrophy of the pancreatic islet. This was also observed in most of these mice at 54 weeks. It was recognized as a continuation of the condition of diabetes mellitus. From the above results, **these mice are considered to be useful as new experimental model animals developing a high rate of obese type 2 (non-insulin dependent) diabetes mellitus** without polyphagia."

Type 2 diabetes mellitus in obese mouse model induced by monosodium glutamate.
Nagata M, Suzuki W, Iizuka S, Tabuchi M, Maruyama H, Takeda SAburada M, Miyamoto K.
Exp Anim. 2006 Apr;55(2):109-15.

"**Administration of monosodium glutamate (MSG) to KK mice during the neonatal period resulted in a syndrome of obesity, stunting and hypogonadism.** In some animals the genetic predisposition to diabetes was unmasked with the development of marked hyperglycaemia and or hyperinsulinaemia. Food intake was not increased compared to controls. The elevated plasma glucose and insulin in fed MSG treated mice fell rapidly with food deprivation. Glucose disposal was comparable in MSG treated and control mice after IP glucose, but after oral glucose MSG treated mice showed impaired glucose tolerance. **Insulin secretion was defective in MSG treated mice.**"

Effects of monosodium glutamate
administration in the neonatal period
on the diabetic syndrome in KK mice.
Cameron DP, Poon TK, Smith GC.
Diabetologia. 1976 Dec;12(6):621-6.

Not all rodent species become obese with MSG ingestion, some just get Diabetes:

Neuronal necrosis in the arcuate and ventromedial hypothalamus regions is easily induced in 1-day-old Chinese hamsters by the administration of monosodium glutamate (MSG). **New-born Chinese hamsters injected with MSG showed no sign of obesity, even when grown up, but apparently developed a diabetic syndrome.**

Diabetic syndrome in the Chinese hamster
induced with monosodium glutamate.
Komeda K, Yokote M, Oki Y.
Experientia. 1980 Feb 15;36(2):232-4.

MSG crosses the Placenta endangering the fetus.

MSG has been shown to cross the placental barrier in rats, and new studies suggest that in cases where human mothers who suffer from intrauterine infection are at risk to Glutamate causing excitotoxic perinatal brain injury to the fetus:

"Monosodium-L-glutamate given subcutaneously to pregnant rats caused acute necrosis of the acetylcholinesterase-positive neurons in the area postrema. The same effect has been observed in the area postrema of fetal rats. The process of neuronal cell death and the elimination of debris by microglia cells proved to be similar in pregnant animals and in their fetuses. However, embryonal neurons were more sensitive to glutamate as judged by the rapidity of the process and the dose-response relationship. **These observations raise the possibility of transplacental poisoning in human fetuses after the consumption of glutamate-rich food by the mother.**"

**Neurotoxicity of monosodium-L-glutamate
in pregnant and fetal rats.**
Toth L, Karcsu S, Feledi J, Kreutzberg GW.
Acta Neuropathol (Berl). 1987;75(1):16-22.

"Monosodium glutamate (MSG) was shown to penetrate placental barrier and distribute almost evenly among embryonic tissues using 3H-Glu as a tracer. When a lower (1.0 mg/g) and a higher (2.5 mg/g) doses of MSG were alternatively injected to Kunming maternal mice in every other days from mating to deliveries, obvious injury occurred in the ability of memory retention and Y-maze discrimination learning of adult filial mice pregnantly treated with higher doses (2.5 mg/g) of MSG. Meanwhile, the neuronal damages were observed in not only arcuate nucleus but also ventromedial nucleus of hypothalamus. Characteristic cytopathological changes induced by MSG showed swollen cytoplasm, dark pyknotic nuclei and loss of neurons.These experimental findings indicated that MSG performed its transplacental neurotoxicity in a dose-dependent manner. The excessive activation of Glu receptors and the overloading of intracellular Ca2+ induced by **MSG ultimately leading to neuronal death may result in the reduction of the capability of learning and memory** in adult filial mice pregnantly treated with MSG."

Transplacental neurotoxic effects of monosodium glutamate on structures and functions of specific brain areas of filial mice
Gao J, Wu J, Zhao XN, Zhang WN, Zhang YY, Zhang ZX.
Sheng Li Xue Bao. 1994 Feb;46(1):44-51.

"Administering GLU to newborn rodents completely destructs arcuate nucleus neurons, and results in permanently elevated plasma leptin levels that fail to adequately counter-regulate food intake. Chronic fetal exposure to elevated levels of GLU may be caused by chronic maternal over-nutrition or by reduced umbilical plasma flow. **We strongly suggest abandoning the flavoring agent monosodium glutamate and reconsidering the recommended daily allowances of protein and amino acids during pregnancy.**"

Does the thrifty phenotype result from chronic glutamate intoxication? A hypothesis.
Hermanussen M, Tresguerres JA.
J Perinat Med. 2003;31(6):489-95

Oral administration of MSG in the pregnant mother's diet has been shown to accumulate at twice the maternal level in the brains of fetal mice:

"Monosodium glutamate (MSG) was shown to penetrate placental barrier and to distribute to embryonic tissues using [3H]glutamic acid ([3H]Glu) as a tracer. However, the distribution is not even; **the uptake of MSG in the fetal brain was twice as great as that in the maternal brain** in Kunming mice. Other maternal mice were given per os MSG (2.5 mg/g or 4.0 mg/g body weight) at 17-21 days of pregnancy, and their offspring behaviors studied. The results showed that maternal oral administration of MSG at a late stage of pregnancy decreased the threshold of convulsion in the litters at 10 days of age. Y-maze **discrimination learning was significantly impaired** in the 60-day-old filial mice."

Effects of maternal oral administration of monosodium glutamate at a late stage of pregnancy on developing mouse fetal brain.
Yu T, Zhao Y, Shi W, Ma R, Yu L.
Brain Res. 1997 Feb 7;747(2):195-206.

In human fetal development, Glutamate is a major contributor to growth of the CNS and brain:

"Glutamate receptors have multiple roles in the central nervous system. Recent evidence suggests that the iontropic **glutamate receptors are critical during brain development**, particularly for corticogenesis, neuronal migration, and synaptogenesis. In this study, we examined subunit mRNA expression and binding sites of the NMDA, AMPA, and kainate receptors from gestational weeks 8-20 in human fetal brain. Expression of glutamate receptors was high during several periods in these brains. These results demonstrate that **glutamate receptors are expressed early in human brain development**."

Ontogeny of ionotropic glutamate receptor expression in human fetal brain.
Ritter LM, Unis AS, Meador-Woodruff JH.
Brain Res Dev Brain Res. 2001 Apr 30;127(2):123-33.

Human fetal development has been shown to be jeopardized by high amounts of Glutamate:

"Children undergoing perinatal brain injury often suffer from the dramatic consequences of this misfortune for the rest of their lives. Despite the severe clinical and socio-economic significance, no effective clinical strategies have yet been developed to counteract this condition. This review describes the pathophysiological mechanisms that are implicated in perinatal brain injury. These include the **acute breakdown of neuronal membrane potential followed by the release of excitatory amino acids such as glutamate** and aspartate. Glutamate binds to postsynaptically located glutamate receptors that regulate calcium channels. The resulting calcium influx activates proteases, lipases and endonucleases which in turn destroy the cellular skeleton. Clinical studies have shown that intrauterine infection increases the risk of periventricular white matter damage especially in the immature fetus. This damage may be mediated by cardiovascular effects of endotoxins."

Perinatal brain damage--from pathophysiology to prevention.
Jensen A, Garnier Y, Middelanis J, Berger R.
Eur J Obstet Gynecol Reprod Biol.2003 Sep 22;110 Suppl 1:S70-9.

"We found evidence that the thrifty phenotype may be the consequence of fetal hyperglutamatemia. Maternal glutamate (GLU) reaches the fetal circulation, as part of the materno-fetal glutamine-glutamate exchange. Glutamine is absorbed from the maternal circulation, and deaminated for nitrogen utilization, resulting in a fetal production of GLU. GLU is extracted as it returns to the placenta. **When the umbilical plasma flow is low, GLU may be trapped in the fetal circulation, and reaches neurotoxic levels.**"

Does the thrifty phenotype result from chronic glutamate intoxication? A hypothesis.
Hermanussen M, Tresguerres JA.
J Perinat Med. 2003;31(6):489-95.

MSG's Ocular Toxicity:

MSG given both subcutaneously and orally in diet causes long term destruction of various ocular structures:

"In rodents, **daily injection of neurotoxic monosodium L-glutamate (MSG) during the postnatal period induces retinal lesions, optic nerve degeneration** with an alteration of visual pathway and an absence of the b-wave in the electroretinogram. Animals received daily doses of glutamate during the first ten days after birth according to two protocols. The two treatments similarly destroyed 56% of the overall population of the ganglion cell layer: 30% of displaced amacrine and 89% of ganglion cells."

Neurotoxic effects of neonatal injections of monosodium L-glutamate (L-MSG) on the retinal ganglion cell layer of the golden hamster: anatomical and functional consequences on the circadian system.
Chambille I, Serviere J.
J Comp Neurol. 1993 Dec 1;338(1):67-82.

"Changes in the transparency and size of lenses in rats were investigated following administration of monosodium-L-glutamate (MSG), MSG (5 mg/g b.w.) was injected subcutaneously on the 9th and 10th days after birth.. The incidence of cataract increased with age, reaching more than 75% at 4 months of age. Morgagni's globules were histologically detected in the opacity of the posterior lens cortex. Degenerative changes of the lens epithelium were observed in the mature cataract. The size and weight of the lens were smaller than those of controls. These findings indicate that **administration of MSG could be an etiologic factor in cataract formation** in the developing rat."

Morphological studies on cataract and small lens formation in neonatal rats treated with monosodium-L-glutamate
Kawamura M, Azuma N, Kohsaka S.
Nippon Ganka Gakkai Zasshi. 1989 May;93(5):562-8.

"The purpose of this study was to investigate the effects of glutamate accumulation in vitreous on retinal structure and function, due to a diet high in sodium glutamate. Three different diet groups were created, consisting of rats fed on a regular diet (diet A), a moderate excess of sodium glutamate diet (diet B) and a large excess of sodium glutamate diet (diet C). After 1, 3 and 6 months of the administration of these diets, amino acids concentrations in vitreous were analyzed. Significant accumulation of glutamate in vitreous was observed in rats following addition of sodium glutamate to the diet as compared to levels with a regular diet. In the retinal morphology, thickness of retinal neuronal layers was remarkably thinner in rats fed on sodium glutamate diets than in those on a regular diet. Functionally, ERG responses were reduced in rats fed on a sodium glutamate diets as compared with those on a regular diet. **The present study suggests that a diet with excess sodium glutamate over a period of several years may increase glutamate concentrations in vitreous and may cause retinal cell destruction.**"

A high dietary intake of sodium glutamate
as flavoring (ajinomoto) causes
gross changes in retinal morphology and
function.
Ohguro H, Katsushima H, Maruyama I,
Maeda T, Yanagihashi S, Metoki T,
Nakazawa M.
Exp Eye Res. 2002 Sep;75(3):307-15.

MSG's Damage to the Liver:

MSG given subcutaneously causes long term destruction of the liver:

"To directly address the long-term consequences of MSG on inflammation, we have performed serial analysis of MSG-injected mice and focused in particular on liver pathology. By 6 and 12 months of age, all MSG-treated mice developed NAFLD and NASH-like histology, respectively. **These results take on considerable significance in light of the widespread usage of dietary MSG and we suggest that MSG should have its safety profile re-examined and be potentially withdrawn from the food chain.**

Monosodium glutamate (MSG): a villain
and promoter of liver inflammation and
dysplasia
.Nakanishi Y, Tsuneyama K, Fujimoto M,
Salunga TL, Nomoto K, An JL, Takano Y,
Iizuka S, Nagata M, Suzuki W, Shimada T,
Aburada M, Nakano M, Selmi C, Gershwin
ME.

J Autoimmun. 2008 Feb-Mar

MSG causes Genotoxicity:

MSG has been shown to be Genotoxic to a variety of organs and tissues in the mammalian body:

Monosodium glutamate (MSG) continues to function as a flavor enhancer in West African and Asian diets. The present study examines the modulatory effects of dietary antioxidant vitamin C (VIT C), vitamin E (VIT E) and quercetin on **MSG-induced oxidative damage in the liver, kidney and brain** of rats. In addition, the effect of these antioxidants on the possible genotoxicity of MSG was investigated in a rat bone marrow micronuclei model. MSG administered intraperitoneally at a dose of 4 mg/g body wt markedly increase malondialdehyde (MDA) formation in the liver, the kidney and brain of rats. The antioxidants tested protected against MSG-induced liver toxicity significantly. VIT E failed to protect against MSG-induced genotoxicity. **The results indicate that dietary antioxidants have protective potential against oxidative stress induced by MSG and, in addition, suggest that active oxygen species may play an important role in its genotoxicity.**

Monosodium glutamate-induced oxidative
damage and genotoxicity
in the rat: modulatory role of vitamin C,
vitamin E and quercetin.
Farombi EO, Onyema OO.
Hum Exp Toxicol. 2006 May;25(5):251-9.

Other Human MSG studies:

MSG connected with adult-onset olivopontocerebellar degeneration:

In patients with recessive, adult-onset olivopontocerebellar degeneration associated with a partial deficiency of glutamate dehydrogenase, the concentration of glutamate in plasma was significantly higher than that in controls. Plasma alpha-ketoglutarate was significantly lower. Oral administration of monosodium glutamate resulted in excessive accumulation of this amino acid in plasma and lack of increase in the ratio of plasma lactate to pyruvate in the glutamate dehydrogenase-deficient patients. Decreased glutamate catabolism may result in **an excess of glutamate in the nervous system and cause neuronal degeneration.**

Abnormal glutamate metabolism in an adult-onset degenerative neurological disorder.
Plaitakis A, Berl S, Yahr MD.
Science. 1982 Apr 9;216(4542):193-6.

MSG connected with amyotrophic lateral sclerosis (ALS):

Glutamate levels were determined in the fasting plasma of 22 patients with early-stage primary amyotrophic lateral sclerosis (ALS) and compared to those of healthy and diseased controls. There was a significant increase (by approximately 100%, p less than 0.0005) in the plasma glutamate of the ALS patients as compared with the controls. Oral glutamate loading (60 mg of monosodium glutamate per kilogram of body weight, taken orally after overnight fasting) resulted in significantly greater elevations in the plasma glutamate and aspartate levels in the ALS patients than in the controls. Glutamate, a potentially neuroexcitotoxic compound, is thought to be the transmitter of the corticospinal tracts and certain spinal cord interneurons. **A systemic defect in the metabolism of this amino acid may underlie primary ALS**.

Abnormal glutamate metabolism in amyotrophic lateral sclerosis.
Plaitakis A, Caroscio JT.
Ann Neurol. 1987 Nov;22(5):575-9.

MSG and the Alteration of the brain: a model for ADHD/Autism

The Erb Hypothesis:

Attention Deficit Disorder, Attention Deficit Hyper Active Disorder, Asperger's Syndrome and Autism are linked. They strike the same percentage of males vs females and have similar characteristic traits. The Erb hypothesis published in 2003 states that Monsodium Glutamate as a food and vaccine additive triggers unchecked brain cell growth. This results in an overgrowth of certain areas of the brain rendering them damaged or destroyed, while accelerating the development of other areas (hence Savants). The genetics and level of MSG exposure determines what level a child will be: ADD, ADHD, Asperger's or Autism.

Autism (or autistic like behaviors) was only known in a handful cases world wide in 1940. ADHD and Autism did not even exist as a diagnosis. In 1950 MSG was introduced to the food supply and the growth of these syndromes has matched the increase in MSG intake in the western diet. As of 2006 there is reported to be one in every hundred children now being born with Autism in the United States.

One of the main characteristics of Autism is a heavier brain. The theory of Mercury causing Autism does not explain the brain overgrowth. Mercury does not enhance cell tissue growth.

In the first 8 weeks of fetal growth the placental barrier is not yet fully formed. This period is when the brain stem, brain, and eyes begin to form.

12 grams a day of MSG in a mother's blood stream could have an enormous affect on the fetal development. Even after the placental barrier has been formed there is not a single human study to show that MSG does not easily transport into the fetus.

Children not born with these ADHD and Autism may have them triggered when an MSG bearing vaccine is injected subcutaneously into them during their formative years.

Accelerated and abnormal brain growth in the Autistic:

Autism most commonly appears by 2 to 3 years of life, at which time the brain is already abnormally large. This raises the possibility that brain overgrowth begins much earlier, perhaps before the first clinically noticeable behavioral symptoms. OBJECTIVES: To determine whether pathological brain overgrowth precedes the first clinical signs of autism spectrum disorder (ASD) and whether the rate of overgrowth during the first year is related to neuroanatomical and clinical outcome in early childhood. Within the ASD group, every child with autistic disorder had a greater increase in HC between birth and 6 to 14 months (mean [SD], 2.19 [0.98]) than infants with pervasive developmental disorder-not otherwise specified (0.58 [0.35]). Only 6% of the individual healthy infants in the longitudinal data showed accelerated HC growth trajectories (>2.0 SDs) from birth to 6 to 14 months; 59% of infants with autistic disorder showed these accelerated growth trajectories. CONCLUSIONS: **The clinical onset of autism appears to be preceded by 2 phases of brain growth abnormality: a reduced head size at birth and a sudden and excessive increase in head size between 1 to 2 months and 6 to 14 months. Abnormally accelerated rate of**

growth may serve as an early warning signal of risk for autism.

Evidence of brain overgrowth in the first
year of life in autism.
Courchesne E, Carper R, Akshoomoff N.
JAMA. 2003 Jul 16;290(3):393-4.

"To establish whether high-functioning children with autism spectrum disorder (ASD) have enlarged brains in later childhood, and if so, whether this enlargement is confined to the gray and/or to the white matter and whether it is global or more prominent in specific brain regions. RESULTS: Patients showed a significant increase of 6% in intracranium, total brain, cerebral gray matter, cerebellum, and of more than 40% in lateral and third ventricles compared to controls. The cortical gray-matter volume was evenly affected in all lobes. After correction for brain volume, ventricular volumes remained significantly larger in patients. CONCLUSIONS: **High-functioning children with ASD showed a global increase in gray-matter,** but not white-matter and cerebellar volume, proportional to the increase in brain volume, and a disproportional increase in ventricular volumes, still present after correction for brain volume."

Increased gray-matter volume in
medication-naive high-functioning children
with autism spectrum disorder.
Palmen SJ, Hulshoff Pol HE, Kemner C,
Schnack HG, Durston S, Lahuis BE, Kahn
RS, Van Engeland H.
Psychol Med. 2005 Apr;35(4):561-70.

"To explore the specific gross neuroanatomic substrates of this brain developmental disorder, the authors examine brain morphometric features in a large sample of carefully diagnosed 3- to 4-year-old children with autism spectrum disorder (ASD) compared with age-matched control groups of typically developing (TD) children and developmentally delayed (DD) children. Cerebellar volume for the ASD group was increased in comparison with the TD group, but this increase was proportional to overall increases in cerebral volume. The DD group had smaller cerebellar volumes compared with both of the other groups. Measurements of amygdalae and hippocampi in this group of **young children with ASD revealed enlargement bilaterally that was proportional to overall increases in total cerebral volume.** There were similar findings of cerebral enlargement for both girls and boys with ASD. In a subgroup of children with ASD with strictly defined autism, amygdalar enlargement was in excess of increased cerebral volume. **CONCLUSIONS: These structural findings suggest abnormal brain developmental processes early in the clinical course of autism."**

Brain structural abnormalities in young children with autism spectrum disorder. Sparks BF, Friedman SD, Shaw DW, Aylward EH, Echelard D, Artru AA, Maravilla KR, Giedd JN, Munson J, Dawson G, Dager SR.Neurology.   2002 Jul 23;59(2):158-9.

Genetic link discovered connecting Glutamate with Autism:

The Autism Genome Project, the largest of its type in research history, found that the genes common among people with ASD (Autism Spectrum Disorder) were ones involved with glutamate :

"Autism spectrum disorders (ASDs) are common, heritable neurodevelopmental conditions. The genetic architecture of ASDs is complex, requiring large samples to overcome heterogeneity. Here we broaden coverage and sample size relative to other studies of ASDs by using Affymetrix 10K SNP arrays and 1,181 [corrected] families with at least two affected individuals, performing the largest linkage scan to date while also analyzing copy number variation in these families. Linkage and copy number variation analyses implicate chromosome 11p12-p13 and neurexins, respectively, among other candidate loci. **Neurexins team with previously implicated neuroligins for glutamatergic synaptogenesis, highlighting glutamate-related genes as promising candidates for contributing to ASDs."**

Mapping autism risk loci using genetic linkage and chromosomal rearrangements.
Autism Genome Project Consortium,

Nat Genet. 2007 Oct

Possible vaccine connection with Autism:

Virus-induced autoimmunity may play a causal role in autism. To examine the etiologic link of viruses in this brain disorder, we conducted a serologic study of measles virus, mumps virus, and rubella virus. Viral antibodies were measured by enzyme-linked immunosorbent assay in the serum of autistic children, normal children, and siblings of autistic children. The level of measles antibody, but not mumps or rubella antibodies, was significantly higher in autistic children as compared with normal children (P = 0.003) or siblings of autistic children (P <or= 0.0001). Furthermore, immunoblotting of measles vaccine virus revealed that the antibody was directed against a protein of approximately 74 kd molecular weight. The antibody to this antigen was found in 83% of autistic children but not in normal children or siblings of autistic children. **Thus autistic children have a hyperimmune response to measles virus, which in the absence of a wild type of measles infection might be a sign of an abnormal immune reaction to the vaccine strain or virus reactivation.**

Elevated levels of measles antibodies in children with autism.
Singh VK, Jensen RL.
Pediatr Neurol. 2003 Apr;28(4):292-4

MSG proven to accelerate the growth of neurons and stimulate proliferation:

"It has been widely accepted that neurogenesis continues throughout life. Neural stem cells can be found in the ventricular zone of the embryonic and in restricted regions of the adult central nervous system, including subventricular and subgranular zones of the hippocampal dentate gyrus. The network of signaling mechanisms determining whether neural stem cells remain in a proliferative state or differentiate is only partly discovered. **Recent advances indicate that glutamate (Glu), the predominant excitatory neurotransmitter in mature neurons, can influence immature neural cell proliferation and differentiation**, as well., Glu can influence proliferation and neuronal commitment as well, and acts as a positive regulator of neurogenesis. Brain injuries like ischemia, epilepsy or stress lead to severe neuronal death and additionally, influence neurogenesis, as well. Glu homeostasis is altered under these pathological circumstances, implying that therapeutic treatments mediating Glu signaling might be useful to increase neuronal replacement after cell loss in the brain."

Glutamate as a modulator of embryonic and adult neurogenesis.
Schlett K.
Curr Top Med Chem. 2006;6(10):949-60.

Evidence of scientific community's awareness that the ingestion of MSG by Humans altered the brain, intelligence and behavior:

The following is a list of published studies for which the main reports are no longer easily accessible. The titles and dates of the studies speak for themselves. The findings of these studies deserve further analysis and should be released to the public. Note: Glutamic Acid is another name for MSG.

The role of glutamic acid in cognitive behaviors; Vogel et. al. 1966.

Glutamic acid and human intelligence; Astin AW, Ross S. 1960

Effects of glutamic acid on behavior, intelligence and physiology. Pallister PD, Stevens RR. 1957

Experimental studies of the effect of glutamic acid-multivitamin combination on the mental efficiency of mentally normal adults. Lienert GA, Matthaei FK. 1956

Effects of prolonged glutamic acid administration on various aspects of personality. Mehl J. 1956

The effects of glutamic acid upon the intelligence, social maturity and adjustment of mentally retarded children. Lombard JP et al. 1955

Glutamic acid therapy in intelligence deficiency. Pabst E, Wurst F. 1952

Improving mental performance with glutamic acid. Kuhne, P. 1951

Glutamic Acid and Intelligence Quotient. Delay J. Pichot P. 1951

An investigation into the effects of glutamic acid on human intelligence. Milliken JR, Standen JL. 1951.

The influence of glutamic acid on test performance. Elson DG et al. 1950.

Effect of glutamic acid on mental function. Kerr W, Szurek S. 1950

Effect of glutamic acid on the intelligence of patients with mongolism. Zimmerman FT et al. 1949.

Conclusions

There are few chemicals that we as a people are exposed to that have as many far reaching physiological affects on living beings as Monosodium Glutamate does. MSG directly causes obesity, diabetes, triggers epilepsy, destroys eye tissues, causes liver damage, is genotoxic in many organs and is the probable cause of Autism. Considering that MSG's only reported role in food is that of 'flavour enhancer' is that use worth the risk of the myriad of physical ailments associated with it? Does the public really want to be tricked into eating more food and faster by a food additive?

MSG is entering our bodies in record amounts with absolutely no limits. The studies outlined in this report often use a smaller proportional dosage than the average child may ingest daily.

A handful of studies prompted an immediate task force on Acrylamide. This report contains dozens of published studies showing proven damage to the mammalian body across a plethora of physiological systems.

Consider the children of the world who eat MSG in their school cafeterias, hospitals, restaurants and homes. They deserve foods free of added MSG, a substance so toxic that scientists use it purposely to trigger diabetes, obesity and epileptic convulsions.

Consider the swift deletion of MSG from the international GRAS lists and the GFSA list of the Codex Alimentarius. Perhaps we will see a reduction in obesity, diabetes, Autism, and many other ailments once the threat to our health from excess Glutamate has been removed.

We can stop the slow poisoning of mankind.

Appendix A List of Foods Approved for MSG Addition

01.1.2 Dairy-based drinks, flavoured and/or fermented (e.g., chocolate milk, cocoa, eggnog, drinking yoghurt, whey-based drinks) 01.3 Condensed milk and analogues (plain) 01.4.3 Clotted cream (plain) 01.4.4 Cream analogues 01.5 Milk powder and cream powder and powder analogues (plain) 01.6 Cheese and analogues 01.7 Dairy-based desserts (e.g., pudding, fruit or flavoured yoghurt) 01.8 Whey and whey products, excluding whey cheeses 02.2.1.2 Margarine and similar products 02.2.1.3 Blends of butter and margarine 02.2.2 Emulsions containing less than 80% fat 02.3 Fat emulsions maily of type oil-in-water, including mixed and/or flavoured products based on fat emulsions 02.4 Fat-based desserts excluding dairy-based dessert products of food category 01.7 03.0 Edible ices, including sherbet and sorbet 04.1.2 Processed fruit 04.2.2.2 Dried vegetables (including mushrooms and fungi, roots and tubers, pulses and legumes, and aloe vera), seaweeds, and nuts and seeds 04.2.2.3 Vegetables (including mushrooms and fungi, roots and tubers, pulses and legumes, and aloe vera) and seaweeds in vinegar, oil, brine, or soy sauce 04.2.2.4 Canned or bottled (pasteurized) or retort pouch vegetables (including mushrooms and fungi, roots and tubers, pulses and legumes, and aloe vera), and seaweeds 04.2.2.5 Vegetable (including mushrooms and fungi, roots and tubers, pulses and legumes, and aloe vera), seaweed, and nut and seed purees and spreads (e.g., peanut butter) 04.2.2.6 Vegetable (including mushrooms and fungi, roots and tubers, pulses and legumes, and aloe vera), seaweed, and nut and seed pulps and preparations (e.g., vegetable desserts and sauces, candied vegetables) other than food category 04.2.2.5 04.2.2.8 Cooked or fried vegetables (including mushrooms and fungi, roots and tubers, pulses and legumes, and aloe vera), and seaweeds 05.0 Confectionery 06.3 Breakfast cereals, including rolled oats 06.4.3 Pre-cooked pastas and noodles and like products 06.5 Cereal and starch based desserts (e.g., rice pudding, tapioca pudding) 06.6 Batters (e.g., for breading or batters for fish or poultry) 06.7 Pre-cooked or processed rice products, including rice cakes (Oriental type only) 06.8 Soybean products (excluding soybean products of food category 12.9 and fermented soybean products of food category 12.10) 07.0 Bakery wares 08.2 Processed meat, poultry, and game products in whole pieces or cuts 08.3 Processed comminuted meat, poultry, and game products 08.4 Edible casings (e.g., sausage casings) 09.3 Semi-preserved fish and fish products, including mollusks, crustaceans, and echinoderms 09.4 Fully preserved, including canned or fermented fish and fish products, including mollusks, crustaceans, and echinoderms 10.2.3 Dried and/or heat coagulated egg products 10.3 Preserved eggs, including alkaline, salted, and canned eggs 10.4 Egg-based desserts (e.g., custard) 11.6 Table-top sweeteners, including those containing high-intensity sweeteners 12.2.2 Seasonings and condiments 12.3 Vinegars 12.4 Mustards 12.5 Soups and broths 12.6 Sauces and like products 12.7 Salads (e.g., macaroni salad, potato salad) and sandwich spreads excluding cocoa- and nut-based spreads of food categories 04.2.2.5 and 05.1.3 12.8 Yeast and like products 12.9 Protein products 12.10 Fermented soybean products 13.3 Dietetic foods intended for special medical purposes (excluding products of food category 13.1) 13.4 Dietetic formulae for slimming purposes and weight reduction 13.5 Dietetic foods (e.g., supplementary foods for dietary use) excluding products of food categories 13.1 - 13.4 and 13.6 13.6 Food supplements 14.1.1.2 Table waters and soda waters 14.1.4 Water-based flavoured drinks, including "sport," "energy," or "electrolyte" drinks and particulated drinks 14.2.1 Beer and malt beverages 14.2.2 Cider and perry 14.2.4 Wines (other than grape) 14.2.5 Mead 14.2.6 Distilled spirituous beverages containing more than 15% alcohol 14.2.7 Aromatized alcoholic beverages (e.g., beer, wine and spirituous cooler-type beverages, low alcoholic refreshers) 15.0 Ready-to-eat savouries 16.0 Composite foods - foods that could not be placed in categories 01 - 15

Appendix B List of Ingredients Containing Glutamate

Always contains MSG:

Monosodium Glutamate
Monopotassium Glutamate   Yeast Extract
Hydrolyzed Protein (any)   Glutamic Acid
Calcium Caseinate   Sodium Caseinate
Yeast Food   Hydrolyzed Corn Gluten
Gelatin   Textured Protein
Yeast Nutrient   Autolyzed Yeast

Often contain glutamate, or create it during processing:

Carrageenan   Natural Pork Flavoring
Citric Acid   Maltodextrin
Bouillon and Broth   Natural Chicken Flavor
Natural Beef flavor   Whey Protein Concentrate
Stock   Whey Protein
Ultra Pasteurized   Soy Sauce
Barley Malt   anything Enzyme
Pectin   anything Enzyme Modified
Protease   Malt flavoring
Protease Enzymes   Soy Protein
Soy Protein Isolate   Soy protein concentrate
Whey Protein Isolate   Malt Extract
anything Fermented   anything Protein Fortified
and even hidden in Natural Flavors & Seasonings

List reproduced with permission from www.Truthinlabeling.org

List from www.truthinlabeling.org

Appendix C List of Vaccines Involving Glutamate

Note: Gelatin and ingredients that use the word Hydrolyzed contain Glutamate.

MMR - Measles-Mumps-Rubella Merck & Co., Inc. 800.672.6372
measles, mumps, rubella live virus, neomycin sorbitol, hydrolyzed gelatin, chick embryonic fluid, and human diploid cells from aborted fetal tissue

M-R-Vax - Measles-Rubella Merck & Co., Inc. 800.672.6372
measles, rubella live virus neomycin sorbitol hydrolyzed gelatin, chick embryonic fluid, and human diploid cells from aborted fetal tissue

Attenuvax - Measles Merck & Co., Inc. 800-672-6372
measles live virus neomycin sorbitol hydrolyzed gelatin, chick embryo

Biavax - Rubella Merck & Co., Inc. 800-672-6372
rubella live virus neomycin sorbitol hydrolyzed gelatin, human diploid cells from aborted fetal tissue

JE-VAX - Japanese Ancephalitis Aventis Pasteur USA 800.VACCINE
Nakayama-NIH strain of Japanese encephalitis virus, inactivated formaldehyde, polysorbate 80 (Tween-80), and thimerosal mouse serum proteins, and gelatin

Prevnar Pneumococcal - 7-Valent Conjugate Vaccine Wyeth Lederle 800.934.5556
saccharides from capsular Streptococcus pneumoniae antigens (7 serotypes) individually conjugated to diphtheria CRM 197 protein aluminum phosphate, ammonium sulfate, soy protein, yeast

RabAvert - Rabies Chiron Behring GmbH & Company 510.655.8729
fixed-virus strain, Flury LEP neomycin, chlortetracycline, and amphotericin B, potassium glutamate, and sucrose human albumin,

bovine gelatin and serum "from source countries known to be free of bovine spongioform encephalopathy," and chicken protein

RotaShield - Oral Tetravalent Rotavirus (recalled) Wyeth-Ayerst 800.934.5556
1 rhesus monkey rotavirus, 3 rhesus-human reassortant live viruses neomycin sulfate, amphotericin B potassium monophosphate, potassium diphosphate, sucrose, and monosodium glutamate (MSG) rhesus monkey fetal diploid cells, and bovine fetal serum smallpox (not licensed due to expiration)

TheraCys BCG (intravesicle -not licensed in US for tuberculosis) Aventis Pasteur USA 800.VACCINE
live attenuated strain of Mycobacterium bovis monosodium glutamate (MSG), and polysorbate 80 (Tween-80)

Varivax - Chickenpox Merck & Co., Inc. 800.672.6372
varicella live virus neomycin phosphate, sucrose, and monosodium glutamate (MSG) processed gelatin, fetal bovine serum, guinea pig embryo cells, albumin from human blood, and human diploid cells from aborted fetal tissue

YF-VAX - Yellow Fever Aventis Pasteur USA 800.VACCINE
* 17D strain of yellow fever virus sorbitol chick embryo, and gelatin

Convenient MSG Ingredient Guide

Permission is granted to reproduce this page for the use of educating and protecting the reader's families and friends.

Always contains MSG:

Monosodium Glutamate
Monopotassium Glutamate   Yeast Extract
Hydrolyzed Protein (any)   Glutamic Acid
Calcium Caseinate   Sodium Caseinate
Yeast Food   Hydrolyzed Corn Gluten
Gelatin   Textured Protein
Yeast Nutrient   Autolyzed Yeast

Often contain glutamate, or create it during processing:

Carrageenan   Natural Pork Flavoring
Citric Acid   Maltodextrin
Bouillon and Broth   Natural Chicken Flavor
Natural Beef flavor   Whey Protein Concentrate
Stock   Whey Protein
Ultra Pasteurized   Soy Sauce
Barley Malt   anything Enzyme
Pectin   anything Enzyme Modified
Protease   Malt flavoring
Protease Enzymes   Soy Protein
Soy Protein Isolate   Soy protein concentrate
Whey Protein Isolate   Malt Extract
anything Fermented   anything Protein Fortified
and even hidden in Natural Flavors & Seasonings

List reproduced with permission from www.Truthinlabeling.org

CPSIA information can be obtained at www.ICGtesting.com
Printed in the USA
LVOW101558190513

334490LV00027B/1160/P